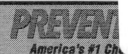

PREVENT
America's #1 Che...

NATURAL
FAT BURNERS

PREVENTION'S BEST™
America's #1 Choice for Healthy Living

NATURAL FAT BURNERS

By the Editors of *Prevention* Health Books

RODALE

ST. MARTIN'S
PAPERBACKS

The information in this book is excerpted from *Banish Your Belly, Butt, and Thighs Forever!* (Rodale, 2000), *Fat to Firm at Any Age* (Rodale, 1998), *Food Smart* (Rodale, 1998), *Maximum Food Power for Women* (Rodale, 2001), *Prayer, Faith, and Healing* (Rodale, 1999), *Prevention's Healing with Vitamins* (Rodale, 1996), *Prevention's Your Perfect Weight* (Rodale, 1995), *The Prevention Get Thin, Get Young Plan* (Rodale, 2001), and *The Woman's Book of Healing with Herbs* (Rodale, 1999).

Prevention's Best is a trademark and *Prevention* Health Books is a registered trademark of Rodale Inc.

NATURAL FAT BURNERS

© 2002 by Rodale Inc.

Cover Designer: Anne Twomey
Book Designer: Keith Biery

ISBN 0-312-98248-8 paperback

Printed in the United States of America

Rodale/St. Martin's Paperbacks edition published October 2002

St. Martin's Paperbacks are published by St. Martin's Press, 175 Fifth Avenue, New York, NY 10010.

10 9 8 7 6 5 4 3 2 1

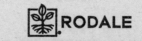

RODALE

WE INSPIRE AND ENABLE PEOPLE TO IMPROVE
THEIR LIVES AND THE WORLD AROUND THEM

Notice

This book is intended as a reference volume only, not as a medical manual. The information given here is designed to help you make informed decisions about your health. It is not intended as a substitute for any treatment that may have been prescribed by your doctor. If you suspect that you have a medical problem, we urge you to seek competent medical help.

Contents

Introduction

This book is written for you—a real person who loves real food. Someone who wants to enjoy many, many more candlelight dinners, listening to her favorite music, while maybe wearing clothes a size or two smaller, and possibly reducing her risk of diseases by as much as half.

Based on the latest research from pioneers in nutritional science, this book translates "what we know" about weight loss into "what to do." Each chapter offers simple fat-burning tips to help you apply these breakthrough discoveries to your life, starting today.

The benefits? Among many others, you'll learn how to:

- Lose weight without obsessing over calories and "forbidden" foods
- Enjoy boundless energy from eating the right food
- Free yourself from rigid diets based on strict "food rules" that don't work (and that cause harm)
- Put binges in their place once and for all
- Fine-tune your vitamin and mineral program to take into account individual differences
- Feast on delicious food while building optimal health
- Harness the slimming power of visualization and prayer

- Build fat-burning muscle and strength through enjoyable exercises and everyday activities

The last point is particularly important. Studies have shown that simple lifestyle changes like taking the stairs instead of the elevator or doing gardening at home are every bit as effective for taking weight off as strict exercise regimens. And they're even more effective at *keeping* the pounds off!

Yes, this book will help you find ways to make exercise and sensible eating enjoyable parts of your day. But it doesn't stop there. It also shows you how to boost your self-confidence and overcome stress—two key elements in maintaining a healthy weight. (Research has found that self-esteem is absolutely crucial for taking off pounds and that stress is the number one obstacle to maintaining a weight-loss program.)

A New You

When you lose weight, the most immediate and often most dramatic benefit is increased energy. You breathe easier. There's less strain on your back and joints. You start to develop a whole new, more active and happier lifestyle.

Let this book start you on the path to a new, happier you. Let it show you that healthy weight loss isn't just a matter of "How much did I lose?" but the powerfully positive "Look what I gained!"

PART ONE

The Eight Keys to Fat-Burning Weight Loss

The First Key: Prepare for Your Journey

For many Americans, trying to lose weight is a national pastime. A Gallup poll reported that 52 percent of Americans are currently dieting or have dieted in the past. One out of six Americans diets each year. A survey of 629 women in a weight-loss registry found that 93 percent of them had unsuccessfully tried to lose weight in the past.

Chances are that you've been down this road before, too. This probably isn't the first time—it might even be the twentieth time. The goal is to make it the *last* time.

How do you do that? With forethought. People often head out on the road to weight loss without first taking the time to figure out whether they are ready and how they will reach their destination.

The real road to a new you starts before you take even a single step. First, take some time to prepare yourself for the journey so that the bad habits you break—and the good habits you make—last a lifetime.

Weight loss—even if it involves fun and simple lifestyle changes—still requires time, dedication, and effort. You have to be ready to make these changes and to give yourself the support you need to succeed.

"In many cases, people are not geared up. And if you are really not ready to go through this, you're not going to be successful," says Ross Andersen, Ph.D., assistant professor of medicine at Johns Hopkins University School of Medicine in Baltimore and one of the nation's leading researchers on lifestyle activity and weight loss.

But how do you determine if you are ready? Try the following:

Weigh the pros and cons. Dr. Andersen asks his clients to write down the benefits and drawbacks of trying to lose weight. For example:

Pros	Cons
Will have a sleeker, healthier body.	Need to get up earlier in the morning to exercise.
Will have more energy; will feel better about self.	Can't go out with the gang every Friday after work to get nachos and margaritas.

"Ask yourself: 'What are the benefits of losing weight right now?' Then compare them with the sacrifices you'll have to make," Dr. Andersen says.

Most times, you'll see that the pros heavily outweigh the cons. And that means you're ready to go. But if it seems to you that the drawbacks outweigh the benefits, he adds, it may mean that this isn't a good time for you to start.

Write out your fears. What are you afraid of if you try to lose weight? Are you afraid that you won't succeed? Or that you won't be able to eat the foods you like? Put these worries on paper.

"When you start to write those things down, they don't have as much power as they did when you kept them secret. It gives you power when you put it down on paper," says Gary Ewing, M.D., director of preventive medicine at the University of South Carolina School of Medicine in Columbia. Not only will they seem less daunting, but in black and white they may even appear unfounded.

Realize that this is a lifetime plan. To be truly ready, you must come to terms with the fact that this isn't a short-term "diet." The changes you are about to make will last for the rest of your life. How do you know when you're ready for this? When you can recognize that this isn't a health kick or fad, says William Smucker, M.D., designer of the Reasonable Eating and Activity to Change for Health program at Summa Health System in Akron, Ohio.

"You have to accept that this is what you eat. This is who you are. This is the way you always intend to do it. The good thing is that the longer one does it, the more likely it is to become a habit," he says.

Sign a contract. Draw up a contract that states that you are committed to giving yourself the time, resources, and energy you need to lose weight, Dr. Ewing says. Sign it, even have someone witness it, and keep it where you'll see it. That way, you'll know that you mean business. If you're willing to sign on the dotted line, you're ready.

"By signing a contract, you say to yourself: 'This is important to me, and I have every intention of following through with this,'" he says.

Preparing for the Journey

Legendary college basketball coach Bobby Knight once said, "The will to succeed is important, but what is more important is the will to prepare." Wise words for losing weight as well. It's wonderful that you want to do it, but that desire is not enough.

After you have decided you're ready, the next step is to prepare for your journey. Just as with those long family vacations, the more you pack, plan, and anticipate those trouble spots during the long trip, the more enjoyable your travels will be.

Here's how to plot your course.

Set a start date and stick to it. How many times have you decided to start a weight-loss program on Monday morning?

By Tuesday afternoon, you realize that you're not ready for this. By Wednesday night, you're off it. And by Saturday, you're saying, "I'll start again Monday." Give yourself some time to prepare. Set a start date, perhaps a week or two down the road, or maybe choose a milestone date, such as a birthday or anniversary, Dr. Ewing says. Then use the time before the start date to get ready.

But take note: Putting off your start date a few days or weeks doesn't mean that you have to eat everything in sight. "A lot of people have what we call the Last Hurrah Suppers," Dr. Andersen says. "That just sends you further back."

Write out your goals. The road to a new you needs a clearly defined route. A road map, if you will. So write out clear-cut, attainable goals. (For more information, see The Fourth Key: Set Realistic Goals, on page 34.) That way, you're saying not only that you want to lose weight but also how you intend to do so. To stay motivated, carry your goals in your wallet or post them in your kitchen or office, Dr. Smucker says.

Watch—and write down—what you eat. A week or two before your start date, begin keeping a food diary. (To learn how, see page 40.) That will help you see what you need to work on before you actually start, Dr. Ewing says. It will help you anticipate potential roadblocks and cut down the odds that you'll go off course in the beginning weeks.

Plan, plan, plan. It may be a week or so before your start date, but now is the time to buy new walking shoes, collect healthy recipes that interest you, throw out the potato chips, stock up on fruits and vegetables, and clear your schedule.

"Look at all the things you have to change, and start to plan out what you have to do," Dr. Smucker says.

If you wait until you start, you'll find yourself staring at an empty refrigerator on your first night, wondering how you're going to make a healthy meal out of chocolate pudding, leftover pizza, and diet soda. Or you'll be inspired to take a walk but won't be able to because your sneakers barely have soles.

Learn from the Past

In 1991, Canadian explorer, adventurer, and inspirational speaker Jamie Clarke was a member of an expedition to climb Mount Everest. He and his team failed, 3,000 feet from the top. Two-and-a-half years later, he tried again to scale the highest point on the planet. When a member of his party became ill, they had to abandon the effort at a distance of just two city blocks from the summit.

The two failed attempts didn't discourage him, though. On his third try, in 1997, Clarke made it to the summit. And he credits his past *failures* for his ultimate success. Clarke studied his previous two attempts and from each one learned how he would do it differently the next time up.

"You have failures, and those failures are the essence, the building blocks, of future success. They are integral. Without them, you cannot have the victory. Because you learn so much from them," he says.

Losing weight can seem as daunting as climbing Everest. But like Clarke, you can use past attempts to fuel your success this time out.

Instead of chalking up previous efforts as part of a long history of unexplainable failures, study, analyze, and learn from them, Dr. Andersen suggests. "What are you going to do differently? Look at and reflect on what led to the collapse of previous attempts," he says.

Setbacks: The Key to Success

Know this scenario? You go on a diet, and you're doing just fine until you find yourself at an office party. Next thing you know, you've swallowed the caloric equivalent of what you'd normally eat in a couple of days. Feeling blue about it, you go home and sulk on the couch, eating a bag of potato chips instead of taking your usual walk. Now that you've really blown it, why bother? You give up entirely, chalking up another failed attempt at losing weight and deciding that it's useless. Then you reach for the ice cream.

The biggest mistake people make while trying to lose weight is that they don't accept their mistakes. They eat one morsel too many or skip one workout, and chuck the whole thing, discarding past successes and throwing aside future victories.

Setbacks aren't the end of a weight-loss effort; they are part of the process, Dr. Ewing says. When you accept this fact of life, you'll continue heading in the right direction even when you take a slight detour. The key is to make setbacks a learning tool, a mechanism that will actually increase your chances of success.

"What are you going to do when faced with these setbacks? Should you go ahead and feel guilty about them, which will cause you distress, and then you'll give up? Or are you going to accept that you will have these lapses and try to learn from each one?" Dr. Ewing says.

Consider each lapse a learning opportunity. Study it. Talk about it. Figure out what went wrong and how to avoid letting it happen again.

"Know that you will relapse. But take comfort in knowing that, and that you'll work on your reaction to these lapses. If you know this going in, it won't be so alarming when it happens. It will just be part of the process," Dr. Ewing says.

The Second Key: Understand Why It's Good for You

Excess weight is bad for you. Of course, you already know that. But exactly how unhealthy is it to carry around extra pounds? The answer, in a word, is *very*.

If you've ever needed to boost your motivation to eat better, exercise more, and peel away that excess poundage, read on.

First and foremost, you should know that being overweight has been directly linked to the leading causes of death in this country today: heart disease, certain types of cancer, stroke, and diabetes. In addition, excess weight is tied to a host of other conditions of varying degrees of severity, ranging from varicose veins to sleeplessness.

In short, the statistics are staggeringly in favor of achieving and maintaining a reasonable weight if you want to live a long, healthy life.

And while the most significant health problems crop up when a person is clinically obese—that is, 20 percent or more above her ideal weight—it doesn't take a big weight loss to effect substantial health improvements. If you have high blood pressure, for example, losing just 10 pounds can help reduce it, say health officials at the Michigan Department of Public Health.

"Look," you may well be saying, "I just want to drop a few pounds because I want to fit into that size 8 dress I have my eye on." That's fine. But just in case you need further incentive to launch a serious weight-loss and -maintenance program, here are some of the main health benefits you'll reap almost immediately after you start to slim down.

Having a Healthier Heart

Each year, more than 900,000 Americans die of heart disease. Almost half of these victims are women. Every year, an additional 1.25 million have a nonfatal heart attack. And nearly one-third of adults suffer from high blood pressure, which can lead to heart disease and stroke. A major cause of all of the above problems is excess weight. Think about it: The more you exceed your recommended weight, the more your heart has to keep pumping to do its job and the greater the pressure you're placing on it.

But if you lose weight, high blood pressure almost inevitably drops. In one study, done at the University of Pennsylvania's Obesity Research Group, people with high blood pressure experienced reductions in blood pressure even in the early stages of their weight-loss diet.

The kinds of foods you're eating will also affect your heart, determining whether your arteries are open and free-flowing or as clogged as a drain begging for Drano. A diet high in fat, particularly the saturated fat that comes from animal sources, causes arteries to plug up with a gooey substance called plaque. Blood has a harder time circulating through plaque-filled arteries. But a diet in which no more than 25 percent of calories come from fat keeps blood flowing smoothly, and dramatically cuts your chances of having a heart attack.

Boosting Good Cholesterol

By now you probably know that LDL, or "bad," artery-clogging cholesterol is affected by the foods we eat—especially the amounts and types of fat. But did you know

Smoke-Free and Chubby?

If you're worried you'll gain weight when you quit smoking, here's what to do.

Keep your mouth busy. Chew on sugarless gum or "smoke" a plastic cigarette. Keep your hands occupied with needlework or gardening or by taking a computer class.

Drink plenty of water. It will aid in digestion and help relieve the bloated feeling ex-smokers sometimes get.

Eat a healthy, balanced diet. If you feel the urge to snack, have cut-up veggies, a handful of thin pretzel sticks, some sugar-free iced tea, or mineral water.

Satisfy your sweet tooth. Try low-fat or fat-free frozen yogurt, fat-free frozen fruit bars, or sugar-free versions of kids' fruit drinks.

Use a food diary. Writing down everything you eat helps you focus on any changes in your eating behaviors.

Exercise. Especially if you tend to be inactive, you'll need to launch a workout schedule—even a modest one—to counteract your now slower metabolism (nicotine increases metabolism). Some ex-smokers report that beginning an exercise program a month or two before they

that you can also increase your HDL, or "good," artery-cleaning cholesterol by losing weight? Regular exercise also helps.

Happily, you needn't wait until you reach your goal weight to see good HDL results. "Even rather small weight losses—10 percent of initial weight or so—will result in increased HDL levels," says F. Xavier Pi-Sunyer, M.D., director of the Obesity Research Center at St. Luke's–Roosevelt Hospital Center in New York City. (An HDL level

plan to quit smoking is easier and ultimately more long-lasting than attempting both simultaneously.

Weigh yourself once a week. The moment you notice a pound or two you didn't notice before, increase your exercise by an extra 30 to 60 minutes a week.

Find a distraction. Start focusing on things other than smoking and eating. Clean out the garage, join a community project, take a workshop in a subject you've always wanted to explore.

Check out a smoking-cessation clinic. Not only will these sessions help you kick your tobacco addiction, but also they'll give you support for dealing with your food cravings.

Give yourself a break. Maybe now's not the time to think about quitting smoking *and* maintaining your weight. After all, kicking the cigarette habit is an achievement in and of itself. If you find yourself gaining 5 or 10 pounds and can't handle the thought of dieting, too, perhaps the smartest thing is to wait until you've been smoke-free for a while and then begin your weight-loss plan again.

of 60 milligrams per deciliter of blood or greater is considered good; at less than 35, it's a risk factor for heart disease. And an LDL reading of under 130 is desirable; it's risky when it hits 160 or above.)

Your cholesterol may rise as you get older, and while you can't do much to avoid birthdays, you certainly can start to lower your cholesterol readings by lowering your weight. "The younger you are and the less fat you carry, the better your chances of reducing your cholesterol levels to well within the desirable range—say, 175 to 195 mil-

What's Up, Doc?

Want to launch a weight-loss program? Consulting your physician for help and advice is a good idea, but don't assume that he necessarily practices what he might preach to you about a healthy diet.

One survey revealed that more than half (55 percent) of U.S. doctors are overweight. And while they may know the value of eating five daily servings of fruits and vegetables, a scant 20 percent do so. A whopping 66 percent confessed that they had eaten some candy "in the past week." The survey was conducted in 1993 by Sudler and Hennessey, the health care and pharmaceuticals advertising division of Young and Rubicam.

"I was surprised that so many physicians said they were overweight," says John Chervokas, the Sudler and Hennessey executive vice president who headed up the survey. "We received a much larger response from doctors than we had originally anticipated, which proved to us that the doctors are interested in the subjects of diet and nutrition. Or maybe they're just interested in food!"

ligrams total cholesterol per deciliter of blood," reports Louis J. Aronne, M.D., associate professor of clinical medicine at New York Hospital–Cornell University Medical College in New York City.

Decreasing the Risk of Diabetes

Of all the major diseases, diabetes is the one most clearly linked to being overweight. Of the 11 million Americans suffering from the disease, 90 percent have non-insulin-dependent (type 2) diabetes—precisely the type most closely associated with excess weight.

"There's no question that obesity is a major contributor to the development of diabetes," says Susan Zelitch Yanovski, M.D., an obesity expert at the National Institute of Diabetes and Digestive and Kidney Diseases in Bethesda, Maryland. But here again, the news is good. "Even a modest weight loss," she says, "can significantly reduce risk for the development of diabetes, as well as improve the blood sugar of those who already have it."

Adds Dr. Pi-Sunyer, "In people with non-insulin-dependent diabetes, blood sugar levels improve within days after starting a weight-loss program, and in some cases medication can be greatly reduced or eliminated."

Preventing Cancer

While there's some debate over whether being overweight is a factor in breast cancer, there is a distinct relationship between breast cancer and a high-fat diet, which generally leads to extra weight as well. In Japan, where until recently fat intake was far lower than ours, the incidence of breast cancer was also far lower.

However, things are changing. As the Japanese eat more fat and their diet begins to resemble the typical, high-fat American diet, they are experiencing more breast cancer.

Many experts now believe that limiting dietary fat to no more than 20 percent of calories consumed—a figure substantially lower than the government's recommended ceiling of 30 percent—is the ideal way to ward off breast cancer. But even if you can't maintain that low a percentage, cutting fat to whatever level you can will still dramatically cut your chances of getting breast cancer, which strikes one in every nine American women.

In addition to breast cancer, overweight women experience greater incidence of other types of cancer, including ovarian and cervical. "Studies have shown that obesity leads to increased levels of estrone, a cancer-promoting hormone," says Dr. Yanovski. "While not all of the evidence for this is clear right now, it is likely that being at a healthy body weight would help give protection from these forms of cancer."

In men, high-fat diets have been associated with prostate cancer, and so they, like women, would be wise to limit their dietary fat intake to no more than 25 or 30 percent of calories from fat.

Living Longer

Again, the Japanese seem to have many of the answers. Despite their unfortunate, and growing, fondness for our own beloved high-fat fast foods, the traditionally low-fat Asian lifestyle generally means a longer life: Japanese men and women have the longest life expectancy in the world.

A new study has also shown that you'll function better as you age if you keep body fat down. Larry Wier, Ed.D., director of the health-related fitness program at the NASA Johnson Space Center in Houston, studied 300

Weight Down, Sex Up

Want yet another good reason to lose weight? It'll give a boost to your sex drive!

Ronette Kolotkin, Ph.D., director of the behavioral program at the Duke University Diet and Fitness Center in Durham, North Carolina, conducted a pair of studies examining the relationship between weight and quality of life. Sixty-four overweight people entering a typical one-month weight-loss program at Duke were asked to respond to statements about how weight affects their quality of life, including six about sexual life.

- "I do not feel sexually attractive."
- "I have little or no sexual desire."
- "I don't want anyone to see me undressed."
- "I have difficulty with sexual performance."
- "I avoid sexual encounters whenever possible."
- "I do not enjoy sexual activity."

A month later, after completing a program of eating right, exercising, and losing weight—on average 8 to 30 pounds—they were asked about the same six statements. To a man (and woman!), they answered quite positively.

"They reported that now they felt more sexual desire and more sexually attractive," reveals Dr. Kolotkin. "What's interesting to note is that someone answering the questions might have lost 20 pounds and still have had 20 or 50 to go. So the point is, you don't need to lose all your excess weight in order to have a quality-of-life improvement—including in your sex life."

women and their ability to use oxygen during exercise. Although it had always been believed that one's exercise efficiency inevitably declines with age, Dr. Wier learned otherwise. "We found that the more body fat a person accumulates over the years, the more of a decline he or she will see," he says. "Some folks over 75 are more functional than others who are much younger. As you grow older, it pays to keep your body fat low and your exercise high."

Fat Hurts More Than Your Looks

A steady diet of fattening foods can take its toll on almost every part of your body, and in ways that won't make you too happy. Here's how obesity can affect you.

Body Part	Problem or Condition
Brain	Stroke
Windpipe	Intensified snoring
Armpits	Excess sweating
Heart	Enlargement, erratic beat, other types of heart disease
Breasts	Cancer
Liver	Cirrhosis
Gallbladder	Gallstones, cancer
Kidneys	Kidney stones, kidney failure due to high blood pressure
Pancreas	Diabetes
Ovaries	Sterility, cancer
Uterus	Cancer
Cervix	Cancer
Hip, knee, and ankle bones	Arthritis
Legs	Varicose veins

Building Better Backs and Joints

Extra pounds up front also invariably lead to extra stress on your back. It's believed that having just 10 too many pounds around your abdomen, centered 10 inches in front of your spine, means your back muscles have to exert a force of 50 pounds to counterbalance your gut.

"Over half of all Americans will eventually develop some back problems, and almost every physician will advise overweight patients with back trouble to reduce their body weight," says Dr. Yanovski.

Doctors also suspect that keeping your weight down will help prevent osteoarthritis by taking a load off your already overworked joints, particularly your knee joints. Nearly 10 percent of folks over 65—and more women than men—suffer from this wear-and-tear knee problem, and obesity is a major risk factor. But if, for example, a 5-foot-4 woman who weighs 165 pounds loses 11 pounds and keeps it off, she can reduce her chances of developing this condition by one-third.

Your hip joints will also thank you if you keep your weight down.

Easing through Pregnancy and Childbirth

The closer you are to your recommended weight, the simpler your pregnancy and delivery will be, says registered dietitian Jo-Ann Heslin, author of 16 books and coauthor of *The Pregnancy Nutrition Counter*. "If you're physically fit, you'll be able to endure labor more easily," she says. "But if you're heavier, you may complicate it, and you'll put yourself at greater risk should you require surgery—the doctor may have to cut through 3 inches of fat before she can get to the baby."

There's no real mystery about delivering a baby, Heslin points out—your body knows how to do it naturally. "But if you're in good shape to start out with, you'll help your body do its job nicely," she says.

Dr. Yanovski adds that an overweight new mom is more likely to develop such complications as pregnancy-induced diabetes and high blood pressure.

"Even though the diabetes usually disappears after delivery, a woman who's had diabetes during her pregnancy must work long and hard to prevent the development of diabetes later in life," she says. "A large number of these women do go on to develop type 2 diabetes."

Getting Well and Staying Well

Any surgery you might need becomes far more difficult and dangerous the heavier you are. But, says Dr. Pi-Sunyer, "just a 10 percent reduction in body weight can reduce the duration of hospitalization and the incidence of postoperative complications."

When you lose weight by cutting fat, you're also giving a big boost to your immune system. That's what scientists at the USDA's Human Nutrition Research Center in San Francisco discovered after monitoring the changes in seven women they studied. Their diets had been reduced from about 41 percent to approximately 30 percent of calories from fat. While this is admittedly a modest study, it suggests that you can only do your immune system good by keeping your weight at a desirable level.

Boosting Energy Levels

Think of how perky you feel when you're lugging home 25 pounds of groceries. Not very? Then you'll have a good idea how an extra 25 pounds (or more) of body weight can drag you down and make you feel more tired and sluggish than necessary. One of the first things dieters report is how much extra energy they have after they've lost even 5 or 10 pounds. They also sleep better.

Many overweight people have a condition known as sleep apnea, and many of those who have it go undiagnosed. Not only do people with apnea snore, but also their breathing passages become blocked. Typically, they wake up again and again or sleep fitfully, never getting adequate rest. "They get drowsy during the day and may start to fall asleep during meetings or while driving their car," explains Dr. Yanovski.

Dieting can help tremendously, she says. "Sleep apnea is very responsive to weight loss."

The Third Key: Determine Your True Weight-Loss Needs

Deciding on a *realistic* new weight is the best way to guarantee that you'll maintain your weight loss and stay thinner for the rest of your life.

For Jill Cude, a 42-year-old engineering company manager from Houston, the weight-loss countdown began one January.

"I wanted to lose weight in time for my 20th high school reunion, scheduled for August," she says. "The question was, how much to take off?"

Jill weighed 143 pounds but longed to return to the lithe 122 pounds she had weighed as a high school senior. "But the dietitian who was helping me suggested that we talk about a more appropriate weight—128 pounds, a weight I could maintain and not look emaciated," she recalls. "At first, I wasn't sure I'd like it."

By August, Jill had shed 15 pounds, reaching her revised but realistic goal. On reunion night, she slipped into a size 6 red silk pantsuit with rhinestones sparkling at the shoulders and discovered that *realistic* also meant attractive. "My outfit looked fabulous," she recalls. "I got a lot of compliments."

Best of all, Jill has maintained her new weight ever since by following a healthy eating plan and fitting lots of activity into her day. Her long-term success is real proof that she had indeed determined her true weight-loss needs. At 128 pounds, Jill looks and feels great, and she can maintain her new slim look with a comfortable amount of physical activity and with meals that don't sacrifice nutrition or the foods she really loves. As a bonus, she has also lowered her risk for a variety of health problems.

Wants, Needs, and Reality

If you've ever stood at the mirror, frowning at your hips, tummy, or thighs, or consulted an "ideal body weight" chart and found that you're pounds away from perfect, then you, like Jill, have probably dreamed about how much weight you *want* to lose.

If a doctor has ever advised you to shed pounds in order to control a medical condition like high blood cholesterol, diabetes, high blood pressure, or heart disease, then you have probably heard about the pounds you *need* to lose.

And if you've ever attempted to slim down and discovered that reaching—or maintaining—a goal weight is more challenging than you ever expected, then it's likely you've discovered that many factors control how much weight you actually *can* lose.

That's why determining your true weight-loss needs is essential. Figuring it out means that you need to balance your desires, your needs, your lifestyle, and your body's natural tendencies, according to Shiriki Kumanyika, R.D., Ph.D., professor and head of the department of human nutrition and dietetics at the University of Illinois, Chicago, and a member of the advisory committee that established the U.S. government's 1995 Dietary Guidelines for Americans.

"There's no magic number," says Dr. Kumanyika. "A woman cannot pick a goal weight off a chart. She has to factor in her own current weight and weight history, her family's health history, her personal health goals, her own eating patterns, and her level of activity. Then she can pick a weight-reduction target that makes sense."

For women, making this highly personal decision often means stepping away from our culture's loud-and-clear message that thinner is better.

"Weight for women is a huge emotional issue," says Debbie Then, Ph.D., a psychologist in private practice in Los Angeles. "Women are valued in society for their looks, while men are more often valued for what they do. So women feel much more pressure, from within and from outside, to be thin. As a result, many women never really appreciate their own unique, beautiful bodies."

Experts suggest asking yourself a couple of key questions.

Why Do You Want to Lose Weight?

At the Duke University Diet and Fitness Center in Durham, North Carolina, program and medical director Michael Hamilton, M.D., asks a simple question of women who want to lose weight: Why?

"The best reason to lose weight is if you feel your weight is in some way negatively impacting your life," says Dr. Hamilton.

"Excessive weight could be jeopardizing your health or interfering with your ability to get up in the morning and have the energy to do the things you want to do. It could be making you feel embarrassed and unwilling to go out socially to the movies or on a hike or to parties," Dr. Hamilton says.

So ask yourself, does your weight interfere with your life—physically, socially, or psychologically? If your answer is yes, consider the reasons. Do you find yourself turning to food to calm stress or soothe difficult emotions? If so, it may be time to break the emotional eating cycle. Do you simply feel too big to take part in activities you enjoy, or do you know that your weight is a health risk? Then a new eating plan and more physical activity may be all you need, says Dr. Hamilton.

Do you find yourself postponing changes you would like to make in your life, telling yourself that happiness, new relationships, new interests, or a different job must wait until you've lost weight? The real barrier may not be your weight at all, says Marcia Hutchinson, Ed.D., a psychologist in the Boston area and author of *Transforming Body Image: Learning to Love the Body You Have.*

"I like to ask women, 'Well, what would be different about your life if you were thinner—how would your relationships change, how would the way you project yourself in the world change, how would the way you care about yourself change, how would the way you feel about yourself as a sexual being change?'" Dr. Hutchinson says. "Getting rid of extra pounds won't change other parts of your life, unless you can also make a change in how you think about yourself."

Start by making a list of the things that you would like to do, or be, "if only" you were thinner, suggests Dr. Then. You may want to feel more attractive, take up a new hobby, or make a job change. Next, make an action plan for achieving those goals—which will include, but not be limited to, adopting a healthy eating plan and adding more physical activity to your day. The process may bring up fears and insecurities, but it can also be very empowering, she says.

What Kind of Shape Are You In, Really?

Often, women approach weight loss by dreaming about the number of pounds they would like to lose, rather than by having a clear picture of how their bodies actually look. If your mental image of your body shape is inaccurate—if, for example, you dislike your hips and thighs because you think they're huge when in fact they're only slightly padded, you may set an unattainable weight-loss goal.

"It's important for a woman to have a realistic sense of her body before beginning a weight-loss program," says Yasmin Mossavar-Rahmani, R.D., Ph.D., assistant clinical professor in the department of epidemiology and social medicine at Albert Einstein College of Medicine of Yeshiva University in New York City. "Otherwise, she may diet unnecessarily or try to lose too much weight."

In a study at a Brooklyn hospital, Dr. Mossavar-Rahmani and other researchers asked 150 female employees—from doctors to laundry workers—to estimate their body sizes. When the researchers compared the women's guesses with accurate measurements, they found that half the women had inaccurate perceptions—believing their bodies were bigger, or sometimes smaller, than they actually were. The less accurate a woman's self-perception was, researchers found, the more likely she was to diet.

One way to find out whether you have a true-to-life mental picture of your own body shape is to make, on an old sheet or taped-together newspaper pages, a life-size drawing of what you think your body looks like. Then lie down on the drawing and have a friend trace your true outline, suggests Dr. Hutchinson. "Women tend to overestimate their body sizes. I've asked women to do this in workshops, and invariably their perception and emotional sense of themselves are bigger than they really are."

If, by doing this exercise, you discover that your mental

image of your body is wildly inaccurate, adjust your weight-loss goals accordingly.

Body Mass Index: Better than a Scale

You can further pin down your "real" size with a measurement tool recommended by weight-loss experts: the body mass index (BMI).

Body mass index is a single number based on a scientific formula that compares your height with your weight. (To determine your BMI, consult the chart "Calculate Your Body Mass Index," page 28.) The result helps predict whether you are at risk for weight-related health problems. Most likely your BMI will fall somewhere between 19 and 32. If you're 5 feet 4 inches, for example, and you weigh 122 pounds, your BMI is 21. But if you're 5 feet 4 and weigh 157, your BMI is considerably higher—27. Dr. Hamilton says the safest range is 20 to 25.

"A BMI of 25 to 30 is overweight," says Dr. Hamilton. "Your risk for health problems like heart disease starts going up. Above 30 definitely puts somebody in the obese category."

What's your healthiest BMI? The answer depends a great deal on your personal and inherited risk for a variety of health problems, including the following:

- Heart disease: If you're at risk for heart disease, a BMI below 22 may be safest, according to Harvard University's ongoing Nurses' Health Study. Among 115,886 women studied for eight years, 605 developed coronary artery disease. Women with BMIs under 21 had no elevated risk; risk rose gradually for BMIs up to 25 and then sharply thereafter.
- Diabetes: Women with BMIs over 28 raise their risk of diabetes, according to the American Diabetes Association.

- Breast cancer: If you have a family history of breast cancer, a BMI below 27 may be safer.
- Other health conditions: With a BMI above 27, your risk rises for conditions such as arthritis, gout, and above-normal levels of cholesterol and triglycerides (blood fats that can increase heart disease risk).

Calculate Your Body Mass Index

To find your body mass index (BMI), locate your height in the left column. Move across the chart (to the right) until you hit your approximate weight. Then follow that column down to the corresponding BMI number at the bottom of the chart.

Your ideal BMI? Between 20 and 25. But each woman's ideal BMI depends in part on her personal

Height	Weight (lb.)						
4'10"	91	96	100	105	110	115	119
4'11"	94	99	104	109	114	119	124
5'0"	97	102	107	112	118	123	128
5'1"	100	106	111	116	122	127	132
5'2"	104	109	115	120	126	131	136
5'3"	107	113	118	124	130	135	141
5'4"	110	116	122	128	134	140	145
5'5"	114	120	126	132	138	144	150
5'6"	118	124	130	136	142	148	155
5'7"	121	127	134	140	146	153	159
5'8"	125	131	138	144	151	158	164
5'9"	128	135	142	149	155	162	169
5'10"	132	139	146	153	160	167	174
5'11"	136	143	150	157	165	172	179
6'0"	140	147	154	162	169	177	184
BMI	19	20	21	22	23	24	25

As a rule, women under age 35 should aim for a BMI of 25 or lower. You may gain weight as you age, and starting with a healthy BMI helps protect you from medical problems, says Dr. Hamilton.

What if your BMI is already outside the "ideal" range? The good news is that a woman can reduce her health

health risks and age. Heart disease, breast cancer, diabetes, and arthritis may be affected by a high BMI. On the flip side, the good news for women with high BMIs is this: You can reduce health risks significantly by losing just enough weight to drop one number from your BMI.

Height	Weight (lb.)						
4'10"	124	129	134	138	143	148	153
4'11"	128	133	138	143	148	153	158
5'0"	133	138	143	148	153	158	163
5'1"	137	143	148	153	158	164	169
5'2"	142	147	153	158	164	169	174
5'3"	146	152	158	163	169	175	180
5'4"	151	157	163	169	174	180	186
5'5"	156	162	168	174	180	186	192
5'6"	161	167	173	179	186	192	198
5'7"	166	172	178	185	191	197	204
5'8"	171	177	184	190	197	203	210
5'9"	176	182	189	196	203	209	216
5'10"	181	188	195	202	207	215	222
5'11"	186	193	200	208	215	222	229
6'0"	191	199	206	213	221	228	235
BMI	26	27	28	29	30	31	32

risks if she loses just 10 to 14 pounds—dropping from, say, a BMI of 30 to a BMI of 28—according to a panel of 20 body-weight experts who gathered for the Roundtable on Healthy Weight, a forum sponsored by the American Health Foundation, in New York City.

Through healthy, low-fat eating and a gentle fitness plan, you can reach and maintain a healthier BMI, says Dr. Hamilton.

Where's the Fat?

Where you're overweight can be just as important as how much you weigh. Women who carry extra fat at the abdomen are at higher risk for weight-related health problems, while fat packed on your hips and thighs poses much less risk (though such fat may be harder to get rid of), says Susan Fried, Ph.D., associate professor of nutritional sciences at Rutgers University in New Brunswick, New Jersey, who studies the links between health and abdominal fat.

Get a clear picture of this fat zone with another measurement tool, the waist/hip ratio. Find yours by measuring your waist at the smallest point and your hips at their widest point. Then divide your waist measurement by your hip measurement. (If your waist is 34 and your hips are 42, for example, your waist/hip ratio is 0.8.) For women, waist/hip ratio over 0.8 indicates an increased risk for diabetes, heart disease, and high blood pressure, says Dr. Hamilton.

Diet, aerobic exercise, and strength training all help burn that excess fat. And the best way to keep track of your progress is an old-fashioned tape measure—or your bedroom mirror, Dr. Hamilton adds.

What about using other body fat measuring devices, such as the calipers and electronic testers available in many gyms, to chart your fat-burning progress?

Determine Your Waist/Hip Ratio

Is your weight increasing your risk for health problems? To find out, don't just step onto the bathroom scale. Measure in addition your waist and hips, and use the following formula to determine your waist/hip ratio—an additional method for assessing health risks, says Michael Hamilton, M.D., program and medical director of the Duke University Diet and Fitness Center in Durham, North Carolina.

1. Measure your waist at its slimmest point.
2. Measure your hips at their widest point.
3. Divide your waist measurement by your hip measurement: _____ (waist in inches) ÷ _____ (hips in inches) = _____ (waist/hip ratio).

If the ratio is higher than 0.8, you may be at higher risk for heart disease, stroke, diabetes, high blood pressure, and possibly even breast cancer, according to Dr. Hamilton. Going from fat to firm can help improve your waist/hip ratio and your overall health profile.

"I tell women it's not worth checking unless they're simply interested," says Dr. Hamilton. "The normal body fat range for a woman is 22 to 28 percent. But most measuring devices are not accurate enough to tell you if you've really changed, so it can be frustrating to check it after a few weeks or months. It's better just to look in the mirror—if it looks like fat, it probably is fat."

What's Your Easy "Maintenance" Weight?

You may find another important clue to your body's natural, healthy weight range by thinking back over your weight history as an adult—or by looking through the back of your closet for the clothes that once fit, says Dr. Hamilton.

Take a look at your past—and think about a weight that has seemed natural for you as an adult. Perhaps you weighed 140 for many years, then suddenly began putting on the pounds. Perhaps your "easy maintenance" weight was a bit higher than that or a bit lower. Regardless of the number, it was a weight that seemed to maintain itself, staying nearly the same whether you ate a little more or a little less or engaged in a little more or a little less physical activity.

"I like to find out what a woman weighed before she started to gain weight in adulthood," Dr. Hamilton says. "I ask if there was a weight she somehow easily maintained for a period of time. If there was, then that's probably a reasonable goal to return to."

One woman, who tipped the scales at nearly 200 pounds, told Dr. Hamilton that she wanted to slim down to 130. But when she told him that she had once maintained a weight of 160 and felt pretty good about it, he encouraged her to set a goal of 160 instead of 130.

If you've always been overweight, you may find useful clues in the weights and body sizes of your own relatives, he says.

"If both parents gained weight at a certain time in their lives, there's probably a strong genetic tendency for their children to gain weight then as well," Dr. Hamilton notes. "That simply means you have to be realistic and careful. Genes may influence 30 to 50 percent of your weight, but you can stay in control through a healthy diet and an exercise program," he adds.

What Can You Do for the Long Run?

Your goal weight should be one you can maintain comfortably for years to come, one that fits into your lifestyle.

"The trick is not only losing weight but also keeping it off," says Richard L. Atkinson, M.D., professor of medicine and nutritional sciences at the University of Wisconsin in Madison and past president of the American Society for Clinical Nutrition. "To do that, you have to come up with a plan you can live with forever."

That means you don't want a crash diet or an extreme exercise program. You want practical, healthy low-fat eating strategies that fit all occasions so you won't have to give up birthday cakes, ice cream in summer, or turkey and stuffing at Thanksgiving. And you want fitness options that suit your lifestyle, budget, and schedule.

Don't skimp on vitamins and minerals. "A woman who maintains a low weight by eating few calories is probably not getting enough of the nutrients she needs for good health and protection from disease," Dr. Kumanyika says.

And avoid roping yourself into an exercise plan that's torture or eats up your precious time. "If your life becomes hell, then your weight-loss goal is not workable," Dr. Hamilton notes. "When someone tells me, 'I maintained my goal weight by eating nothing but broccoli three times a day and running 6 miles every morning,' I suspect she's not going to be able to keep it up, because that doesn't sound like a workable lifestyle over the long term."

The Fourth Key:
Set Realistic Goals

Many of us dream of getting back to a weight or clothing size that we associate with a special time in our lives. It's human nature. "After all," the thinking goes, "I was there once, so I can get there again."

What's wrong with this reach-for-the-stars attitude? It undercuts your efforts before you even start, says Ross Andersen, Ph.D., assistant professor of medicine at Johns Hopkins University School of Medicine in Baltimore and one of the nation's leading researchers on lifestyle activity and weight loss.

After repeatedly setting—and missing—these pie-in-the-sky goals, you may give up on weight loss altogether. "When you fail at too many goals, you give up setting goals," says Dana G. Cable, Ph.D., professor of psychology at Hood College in Frederick, Maryland.

This doesn't mean you shouldn't set goals; just make them realistic. With an attainable goal constantly on your horizon, you're always motivated to better yourself. "Goals give us something that is a little out of reach, where we have to commit ourselves," Dr. Cable says.

Goal setting also is a key to staying young, Dr. Cable says. When you know that new benchmarks and successes await you in the future, you'll continue to strive, learn new things, accomplish new goals, and see yourself with a lot more to do in life—no matter how old you are.

Realistic goal setting takes the dreaded failure cycle and turns it completely on its ear. You set short-term, within-reach goals. You achieve those goals, and you feel good about yourself, so you set new goals. Next thing you know, you're tackling goal after goal. And losing pound after pound.

The Gold Standard of Goals

Anyone can dream up an arbitrary goal, but good goals require thought, planning, and creativity. Properly set goals map out the road to get there as well as the final destination.

"A goal without a plan is likely to fail," says Raymond C. Baker, Ph.D., a clinical psychologist and director of the Center for Wellness and Counseling at Bradley University in Peoria, Illinois. So when establishing your weight-loss goals, you should make sure they contain the following vital characteristics.

They are specific, yet flexible. A goal of "I will exercise this week" is too nebulous. It doesn't give you parameters of how or when you will accomplish it, Dr. Baker says. Instead, be as specific as possible so that you give yourself a plan as well. For example, a good goal would be: "I will walk for 30 minutes, 5 days this week, during my lunch hour or right after work."

Just be sure to allow yourself some flexibility. If you could walk only 20 minutes or you had to skip a day, don't feel that you have failed, Dr. Baker adds. Just because you don't always meet your exact goal doesn't mean that you should abandon the effort.

They are reasonable and attainable. If you haven't been exercising lately, a goal of walking 10 miles a day every day of the week is not realistic. If you can't picture yourself doing it, chances are that you can't do it, Dr. Baker says. That's not to say that you can't work up to it, but to go for it right off the bat will doom you to failure. Set goals such as "I'll walk a mile 4 days this week." Once you've mastered this goal, then step it up a notch.

They are measurable. Here's a commonly heard goal: "I'll eat healthier." But just how do you know if you have met that goal? You must be able to evaluate and quantify your success. Set goals that you can count or mark off as you accomplish them, such as getting 30 grams of fiber every day, eating nine servings of fruits and vegetables, walking for 30 minutes, or trying one new food every week, says Dr. Baker.

They can be tracked for progress. By recording your development, you'll see how you are improving and changing. That in itself provides positive feedback and reinforcement, giving you the encouragement you need to keep going, Dr. Baker says. Writing down your progress also allows you to see when you've accomplished one goal and when it is time to reevaluate and move on to others.

Playing the Numbers Game

When measuring your weight-loss goals, the scale should not be your only guide. Use other criteria for success, such as how your clothing fits, how you feel, and what your fitness level is. The scale places too much emphasis on a number, experts say.

While that all certainly is sound advice, the reality is that most of us who are trying to lose weight consider the scale to be the ultimate measure. Chances are that you have—or want to set—a goal weight. So if you are going to do it, do it right.

When picking a goal weight, people tend to make one of two mistakes. Either they pick a weight they have to torture themselves to get to, or they have a lot of weight to lose, so they pick a daunting, long-term weight-loss goal—such as 50 pounds or more.

In the first case, Dr. Andersen says, even those who make it to their target weight find that they can't stay there. "It's one thing to diet down to a certain weight. Some people, however, can't keep it there, but they still think that is their ideal weight," he says. In the second case, setting a goal that seems so far away can overwhelm people before they even begin. "That's part of a big problem. They say, 'I have so much to lose—I don't know how to get started.'"

That's why Dr. Andersen has developed a strategy for choosing a weight-loss goal. It takes into account both common mistakes. It allows you to lose a reasonable amount of weight that you'll be able to maintain. Also, it breaks a major weight-loss goal down into smaller pieces, making it seem much less daunting. Here's how to choose a weight-loss goal that you can reach—and maintain.

Go to the 5 and 10. Reaching a weight-loss goal of 5 to 10 percent of your total weight is considered a huge success. Even if you want to lose much more, start with this goal, Dr. Andersen says. With this percentage, you'll see health and appearance differences, but it isn't so drastic a goal that it is unattainable or unmanageable. So if you are 160 pounds, your initial goal will be between 8 and 16 pounds.

Strive for 1 to 2 pounds a week on average. A slow, steady weight loss is not only healthier but also easier to keep off, Dr. Andersen says. Rapid weight loss, on the other hand, is usually done through drastic measures, so once you go back to your old habits, the weight returns as quickly as you lost it.

Make the lifestyle changes recommended in this book, and you should shed 1 to 2 pounds a week. Just keep this in mind, he advises: Think about it on average over the course of time, instead of worrying about how many pounds you lost in one particular week. One week you may only lose 1 pound, but the next week you could lose 3.

Keep it off for a while. Once you reach your 5 to 10 percent goal, your next goal should be maintaining your new weight, Dr. Andersen says. For many, keeping the weight off is the real challenge. By spending a few weeks or months simply staying at your new weight, you give your body and yourself a breather from the mental and physical rigors of trying to lose weight.

This maintenance period also allows you to make sure that lifestyle changes become just that—permanent changes that you'll carry with you for the rest of your life, not just changes you made for short-term weight loss.

Reevaluate your goal. As you stay in your maintenance phase, think about your next goal. After achieving your initial weight loss, your ideas about how much weight you want to lose and can lose may change. Also, think about what is going on in your life. If it is a hectic time, maintaining your weight for a longer period of time may be more realistic than trying to lose more, Dr. Andersen says.

Strive for another 5 to 10 percent. If you decide to lose more weight, stick to another 5 to 10 percent, Dr. Andersen says. Breaking it down into 5 to 10 percent chunks is more effective than trying to lose a large amount in one shot. "Most people who have significant weight loss do it in chunks. They slice it up a bit."

Making Change

You don't lose 20 pounds just because you want to. "You must exhibit certain attitudes, beliefs, and behaviors that will lead to weight loss," Dr. Baker says.

To do that, you have to set what Dr. Baker calls process goals. These are things you do that lead to weight loss. "You want goals on how to reduce the fat in your diet, increase the amount of fruits and vegetables. These aren't even weight-related. But if you accomplish them, the weight will come off."

Homing in on behavioral goals will help you keep the weight off. And the best way to do that is to focus on specific lifestyle changes. "Try not to make weight loss the goal. Make the behavioral changes the goal. I tell my clients that the weight loss is a fringe benefit," says Lisa Tartamella, R.D., a nutrition specialist at Yale–New Haven Hospital in Connecticut.

Process goals differ from one person to the next—it depends on what you need to work on. To get a good idea of what your behavioral goals should be, keep and study a weight-loss diary, Dr. Baker says. But here are some ideas of process goals that you could set.

- Walk for 30 minutes, five times a week.
- Read a book instead of eating when bored.
- Use your food diary every day this week.
- Bring fruit to work for a snack.
- Try one new fruit, vegetable, or grain each week.
- Schedule 15 minutes each day to just sit and relax.
- Try a new sport or activity once every 2 weeks.
- If you did not meet your goals today, start fresh again tomorrow instead of calling it quits.

The Fifth Key: Keep a Written Record

You already know about the two cornerstones of weight loss: eating right and exercising. But now you need to add a third component that is scientifically proven to take off the pounds: writing.

"When I get a new person in my program, I show them the data on weight-loss diaries, and I just tell them right up front, 'You need to be willing to do this.' Every good weight-control program stresses the importance of self-monitoring. It causes the changes that lead to weight loss and control," says Raymond C. Baker, Ph.D., a clinical psychologist and the director of the Center for Wellness and Counseling at Bradley University in Peoria, Illinois.

Study after study has shown that keeping track of eating and exercise is the key to losing weight and keeping it off. Here are some of the highlights.

- A group that kept detailed food diaries during a 10-week study lost 64 percent more weight than a group that didn't.

- Out of 10 ways to alter eating habits, self-monitoring was the only one that allowed people to keep the weight off for up to 1½ years, one study found.
- In another study group, 89 percent of the people who were able to maintain their weight loss relied on record keeping.
- Two studies have shown that people who consistently self-monitored lost more weight than those who only kept track less than half the time. Only those who self-monitored consistently lost a significant amount of weight.

The reason for this phenomenal success is that people often are unaware of their own behaviors. They get so wrapped up in their day-to-day lives that they don't notice the habits they develop that hamper weight-loss efforts. Because they never identify these problems, they never get the opportunity to fix them.

A weight-loss diary acts as a mirror. Through it, you get a true picture of yourself, your eating patterns, and your exercise routines. You clearly see what you do right, what you need to modify, what works, and what doesn't, Dr. Baker says. It awakens people to their own habits and behaviors and gives them the power to make positive changes.

"It puts you in charge. It gives you the information you need to figure out what works for you. Through self-monitoring, you hit upon a successful eating and exercise plan," Dr. Baker says.

More Than Just Record Keeping

Your weight-loss journal can be more than just the nuts and bolts of your eating and exercise routine. If you want, it can be a source of inspiration, comfort, and relief. Writing may help you unleash what's on your mind, enabling you to lose weight as well as what might be weighing you down. By doing so, it can help you feel younger both physically and mentally, says Howard J. Rankin, Ph.D., psychological advisor to the TOPS (Take Off Pounds Sensibly) Club and author of *Seven Steps to Wellness*. Here are just a few of the other benefits of keeping a weight-loss journal.

Increases accuracy. There's an old Chinese proverb that says, "The palest ink is better than the best memory."

The Secret to Holiday Weight-Loss Success

For even the strongest-willed person, the holidays can prove to be an unforgiving weight-loss nemesis. Surrounded by good food, good drink, good fun, and not much time to exercise, many throw their hands up in defeat and concede that they'll pack on 5 to 10 pounds between Thanksgiving and New Year's Day. If only there was some secret to ward off those unwanted pounds.

Well, now there is. And it's something you should already be doing: Stick with your weight-loss journal.

Raymond C. Baker, Ph.D., a clinical psychologist and director of the Center for Wellness and Counseling at Bradley University in Peoria, Illinois, asked people in a weight-loss program to keep diaries during the holidays.

Those who stayed on track and kept extremely diligent food and activity journals actually lost weight between Thanksgiving and New Year's Day.

"It keeps people focused on their goals and improves their decision making," Dr. Baker says.

With all you have to remember during the day, it's easy to forget the cookies you ate at 3:00 P.M. or the fact that you didn't take your daily walk.

And it's those little things you forget that add up and often make the most difference in your weight-loss efforts. Writing it down guarantees an accurate record, says Dr. Rankin.

Provides clarity and resolution. You may decide that you want your diary to be a daily journal as well. Writing out stressful events or problems often allows you to work through them.

"Writing is thinking. When you start to write something down, you are really crystallizing thoughts and feelings," Dr. Rankin says.

Reminds you of your goals. Not only should your daily diary chronicle what you have done; it should also contain what you want to do. Write down daily, weekly, and long-term goals, says John P. Foreyt, Ph.D., director of the Behavioral Medicine Research Center at Baylor College of Medicine in Houston and coauthor of *Living without Dieting*. Each time you open it, you'll be reminded of what you are striving for.

Motivates you. Your diary will map out your progress. You'll see how far you've come in changing your eating habits, how you've increased your exercise, and how you've met certain goals. It's tangible evidence of your success that you can revisit for inspiration.

"It can be self-rewarding and reinforce what you are doing," Dr. Foreyt explains.

The Write Stuff

There are all kinds of ways to keep a weight-loss diary: Write it down in a notebook, buy a published food and activity log, jot down notes on paper and then transcribe them into a computer file. It doesn't matter how you do it, as long as it works for you, Dr. Baker says.

However you choose to do it, here are some guidelines to ensure that your journal contributes to your weight-loss success.

Make it your constant companion. When Dr. Baker sees food and coffee stains all over someone's diary, he knows that person is doing it right.

"I want that diary to be out there in the battlefield. I don't want a nice, clean diary," he says.

Keeping Track

Based on his published studies and clinical experience, Raymond C. Baker, Ph.D., a clinical psychologist and director of the Center for Wellness and Counseling at Bradley University in Peoria, Illinois, has identified specific details that people need to write down in order to develop a successful weight-loss plan. These questions will construct your weight-loss diary and allow you to discover what you need to do to become thinner and younger. They make you think about much more than what you eat—they address when you eat, why you eat, and how you feel when you exercise.

Depending on how you decide to keep your weight-loss diary, write these questions in your journal or photocopy this page and tuck it away in your diary.

Food
- What did you eat?
- How much? (Record your portion sizes)
- How many calories?
- How many grams of fat?
- What did you drink?
- What time did you eat?

Your journal should be compact enough that you can carry it with you at all times. Look for a notebook or journal that will easily fit in your handbag or jacket pocket. If it isn't with you, you're more likely to forget important details or not maintain the diary at all.

Write it down immediately. Whip out your diary after each meal and after exercising. Why? Because recording your actions immediately helps you plan for the rest of the day, Dr. Baker says.

For instance, say you've had a high-fat meal for lunch.

- How fast did you eat?
- Were you hungry? If you weren't, why did you eat?
- Where were you? What were you doing?
- What emotions were you feeling?
- Did something other than hunger trigger your eating?
- Did you snack?
- What are your dietary goals—and were they met? (For example, amount of fiber, number of servings of fruits and vegetables, glasses of water per day)
- Did you try new foods or ways of preparing foods? Did you like them?

Exercise
- What activity?
- Was it a new activity? Did you enjoy it?
- How long (minutes, hours) or how many repetitions and sets?
- At what intensity did you exercise? (High, medium, low)
- How did you feel afterward?
- If you skipped exercise, why?

By writing it down soon after, you note that you'll have to plan a healthier dinner to offset your lunch. "It allows people to problem solve and make changes that will help their behaviors," Dr. Baker says.

Remember the little things. That pat of butter on your bread, the nibbling you do while making dinner, the three or four cookies you grabbed during your coffee break—these little things add up to pounds over time, Dr. Baker says. And it's these little things that are sometimes the most important to record.

A study at a clinical nutrition center in Cambridge, England, found that people who didn't accurately record their daily intakes of food in their food diaries were overlooking snacks eaten between meals. To get a true picture of your eating habits, you must write everything down, Dr. Baker says.

Be honest. "What I most keenly wish is not to forget that I am writing for myself alone. Thus I shall always tell the truth, I hope, and thus I shall improve myself," said French artist Eugène Delacroix in the opening page of his diary back in 1822. Take the painter's words to heart. This diary is for your eyes only, so don't feel that you have to fudge or hide something you did. There's no reason to be embarrassed by your actions. By being honest and writing them down, you're taking the first step toward making a positive and successful change.

Time to Review

What to do with the mountain of information that you're recording in your diary? Study it, Dr. Baker says. For inside the pages of your diary lies the map to your weight-loss goals. Your evaluation will reveal your own personal weight-loss strategy—a program for you, by you.

Here's how to transform your writing into action.

Analyze weekly. Pick a day—maybe each Sunday—when you look over your diary.

"A week's time is more meaningful, and you'll get a general idea of the trends," Dr. Baker says. Study your goals and results as a weekly measure.

For instance, don't study how much fiber you ate by the day. If you had a bad day, you could get discouraged. Yet if you add up your grams of fiber over the course of the week and divide by 7, you may realize that you did very well on average.

Look for triggers. Scan your diary and look for trends. Did you overeat every time you felt stressed-out? Do you always blow off exercise because you feel tired? Does watching TV automatically send you to the refrigerator? Do you always eat on the run, barely tasting your food? These are the connections you want to discover, suggests Dr. Baker.

Search for successes, too. A weight-loss diary chronicles what works as well as what doesn't, says Dr. Baker. If you notice that you lost weight the week you tried a new exercise or changed an eating habit, you have discovered an effective weight-loss tool for you.

"Losing weight is very individualized, and this will help identify what works for you," he says.

Change your criteria periodically. The goal of this weight-loss diary is to help eliminate bad habits and develop good ones, Dr. Baker says. If you've mastered a behavior such as drinking enough water or walking every day, drop it from your diary. Then concentrate on new goals or other habits that you'd like to break.

The Sixth Key:
Binge-Proof Your Eating

Binges flare up when your resistance is down. To boost your binge "immunity," practice HALT—never get too Hungry, Angry, Lonely, or Tired.

Like tornadoes, binges seem to strike out of the clear blue sky, leaving in their wake cookie crumbs, empty Fritos bags, and guilt.

But is a binge really the irresistible force it seems to be? "Not at all," says Gerard J. Musante, Ph.D., director of Structure House Center for Weight Control and Lifestyle Change in Durham, North Carolina. "Controlling your impulse to binge—and it can be controlled—comes down to how you choose to act." In other words, your behavior.

But before you can change your behavior, you must confront your feelings, says Dr. Musante. You may find that negative emotions—anger, depression, anxiety—are driving your binges.

Once you've made the feeling/food connection, you can work on changing your response to it. The turning point comes when you realize that you have a choice not to pig out. That's when you learn to think through your impulse to eat, then choose whether or not to give in. Then *you* control a binge, not the other way around.

Each time you manage to resist the urge to eat, you create an "I can" moment. "That's when you're hit with the impulse to eat, and you think 'I can handle this,' rather than 'I can't stand it,'" says Lee Kern, a licensed clinical social worker and clinical director at Structure House. "That's a very powerful moment."

To avoid a binge, use the first through fourth commandments, below. To stop one already in progress, use the fifth through seventh commandments. To bounce back from a binge, turn to the eighth through 10th commandments.

Commandment #1:
Thou Shalt Not Set Thyself Up

Stop berating yourself: You don't pig out because you lack willpower or self-control. "Women think binges fall out of the sky," says Kern. "The truth is, many women set themselves up."

The biggest unconscious setup is poor time or lifestyle management. Long, seemingly endless days bereft of friends or meaningful activity can send you straight to the fridge. "For these women, a binge becomes the pleasure and entertainment of the day," says Kern.

Those who juggle a multitude of obligations—houses, spouses, kids, and career—may use eating everything that isn't nailed down as a way to spend some time alone after a day of being a caretaker. To stop the setups, analyze the ways in which you manage your time and your life, recommends Kern. Do you have too little time for yourself—or too much? Do you take time to relax and regenerate? Are some of the obligations in your life self-imposed, and

Define a Binge

How many doughnuts make a binge? Three, if you're a woman. Six, if you're a man, according to a survey of 400 college students.

might dropping them make your life less hectic? Once you've answered those questions, you can generate solutions.

If you have too much time on your hands, take steps to fill it with activities other than eating. Take classes, sign up for volunteer work, or made a standing daily date for a brisk walk with a friend. If your impulse to eat arrives at a certain time—say, 11:00 A.M., 3:00 P.M., or right after work—schedule your chosen activity during this time.

If your family and job leave you overextended, announce to your family that from now on you'll be taking a 30-minute breather when you get home or at another specific time. Then head for a bubble bath, the home gym, or a juicy novel.

Commandment #2: Thou Shalt Not Starve Thyself

Many women, having eaten too much at dinner, feel they have to atone for their extra calories. "So they skip breakfast and lunch the next day," says Shannon Turner, Ph.D., professor of clinical health psychology at the Oklahoma State University College of Osteopathic Medicine in Tulsa.

Big mistake. "All skipping meals does is make you famished—which may push you right into a binge," says Dr. Turner.

Another pitfall is being too busy to eat breakfast or lunch, then arriving home at the end of the day hungry enough to gnaw your kitchen cabinets. If you're a meal skipper, eating three meals a day—including breakfast—will ensure that you never get too hungry.

If your stomach lurches at the very thought of eating in the morning, start small, perhaps with a piece of whole wheat toast and a teaspoon of peanut butter or with a carton of low-fat fruit yogurt. If you dislike traditional breakfast fare, opt for half a sandwich—like thin-sliced deli ham and reduced-fat cheese on a piece of whole grain bread.

If it's hard for you to sit down to three meals, try eating every 3 to 4 hours (roughly five or six mini-meals each day), suggests Dr. Turner. "Some women find that small, frequent meals help them curb their urge to binge."

As often as possible, make mealtime an event. Eat at the kitchen or dining room table, rather than in front of the TV. Eliminate distractions. "Put the magazine down, put away your work, hang up the phone," says Dr. Turner. At work, if you eat lunch at your desk, put away your paperwork and put your phone on private.

Commandment #3: Thou Shalt Strip Thy Trigger Foods of Their Power

Every woman knows her trigger food like she knows her Social Security number. It's the one she can't put down until she's demolished the entire package. (Call it the you-can't-eat-just-one syndrome.)

Often, trigger foods are what Dr. Musante calls primary foods—those you've learned to associate with feelings of comfort, security, or happiness, sometimes before you even learned to talk.

Yet you can learn to recreate the positive feelings that

trigger foods evoke—without the food itself, says Dr. Musante. He suggests the visualization below.

Think back to your earliest memory of your trigger food—say, potato chips. Perhaps you first remember enjoying these salty rounds at the age of 5 or 6, at a family picnic by the lake.

Close your eyes and remember the scene. But edit out the chips.

When a Carrot Doesn't Cut It

Trying to white-knuckle a craving can put you on the fast track to a binge, says Catherine Christie, Ph.D., president of Nutrition Associates in Jacksonville, Florida, and coauthor of *I'd Kill for a Cookie*.

Her advice? Either feed your craving—in moderation—or choose foods that can stand in for the creamy, crunchy, or greasy sensations your tastebuds demand. Here's a short list of substitutes that satisfy.

When You Want Chocolate
- 1 tablespoon of chocolate chips (27 chips: 70 calories, 4 grams of fat)
- Four Hershey's Kisses (105 calories, 3.8 grams of fat)
- 4 ounces of Snack Pack fat-free chocolate pudding (98 calories, zero gram of fat)

When You Want Salty Snack Foods
- 36 Guiltless Gourmet corn tortilla chips (try the chili and lime or Mucho Nacho) and salsa (220 calories, 4 grams of fat)
- Six cheese or nacho cheese mini rice cakes (53 calories, 0.5 gram of fat)
- 33 mini pretzels (52 calories, zero gram of fat)

Now you're free to focus on the scene itself. Conjure up its sights, sounds, sensations. The sound of your brother's splashing. The warmth of the sun on your hair. The laughter of your parents from the lake as you lay on the soft grass, watching the clouds. Feel the comfort of that scene, when all your needs were automatically met, when you were carefree.

Hold that image until you're smiling with your eyes closed.

When You Want Cookies, Cake, or Pie
- Low-fat whole grain cereal bar (136 calories, 2.8 grams of fat)
- 2-ounce slice of angel food cake (73 calories, 0.2 gram of fat) topped with fresh raspberries
- 1-ounce slice of pound cake (131 calories, 7 grams of fat) topped with fresh sliced strawberries
- 7 ounces of light cherry cheesecake yogurt (130 calories, 1.5 grams of fat)

When You Want Ice Cream
- ½ cup of frozen yogurt topped with 1 tablespoon of fat-free caramel topping (165 calories, 4.3 grams of fat)
- ½ cup of vanilla ice milk topped with 1 tablespoon of fat-free hot fudge topping (142 calories, 3 grams of fat)

When You Want Fast Food
- Small hamburger (231 calories, 8.6 grams of fat)
- 20 to 25 french fries (235 calories, 12.2 grams of fat)
- Chicken wing or drumstick (140 calories, 10 grams of fat)

See? You've drawn the comfort you needed from memory alone. You didn't need the chips to take you there.

Commandment #4:
Thou Shalt Give Thyself Regular Tune-Ups

Many of us are religious about taking our cars in for their tune-ups, the idea being that it's better to head off problems before they occur.

Use the same principle with yourself, says Kern. If you don't want to drive yourself into the ground, you need to schedule regular "tune-ups" that nourish you in ways that don't involve food.

Take 10 minutes to develop a list of daily, weekly, and monthly tune-ups, advises Kern. "The list of one woman I worked with read something like this: 'Every day, I need to spend at least 15 minutes in inspirational reading. Every week, I need to make an appointment to get my hair done. And every month, I need to spend a weekend in the city alone to go to the symphony and hit the museums.'"

Develop and write your list, adds Kern. Find a quiet 15 to 20 minutes—before bed, perhaps, or in the morning. Hang the list in a prominent place—on the edge of your bedroom mirror, maybe. You can even put your tune-ups on your home or work computer's scheduling software. (If you'd rather not advertise your list, laminate it and carry it in your purse. Pull it out when you first feel a binge coming on.)

Feel guilty about your tune-ups? Look at it this way. You already feel guilty about bingeing. Moreover, you're unlikely to stop until you find more positive ways to nurture yourself.

"You have to say, 'These are the things that make me feel good about myself. And if I don't do them, then I'm setting myself up for a binge,'" says Kern.

Do You Have Binge-Eating Disorder?

Imagine eating a large pizza, three cheese sandwiches, a pint of ice cream, and five pieces of cake—all within 90 minutes.

This isn't the face of gluttony. It's the face of a binge-eating disorder (BED), thought to affect up to two million Americans—60 percent of them women. Experts aren't sure what causes BED, but up to half of all people with the disorder have a history of depression.

Only a specialist can tell you whether your overeating might signal BED. But women diagnosed with this condition:

- Have binged at least twice a week for at least 6 months
- Eat abnormally large amounts of food in a short period of time
- Eat much more quickly than normal
- Eat until they're uncomfortably full
- Eat alone because they're embarrassed by how much they eat
- Find that they can't stop eating, even if they want to
- Feel disgusted, depressed, or guilty about their binges

For more information on BED, including where to find treatment in your area, call Eating Disorders Awareness and Prevention, a Seattle-based nonprofit organization devoted to bringing BED and other eating disorders out of the shadows. The toll-free number is (800) 931-2237. You can also get more information through the organization's Web site at www.edap.org.

Commandment #5:
Thou Shalt Not Eat around a Craving

We've all done it. Confronted by a Grand Canyon craving for sour-cream-and-onion potato chips, we resist. Instead, we make do with three pieces of buttered toast, half a box of dry breakfast cereal, and most of the kids' fruit rolls.

Eat the chips, already.

When you resist a craving, you often eat everything else in sight. "That's called eating around a craving," says Catherine Christie, Ph.D., president of Nutrition Associates in Jacksonville, Florida, and coauthor of *I'd Kill for a Cookie*. "I've had clients who craved chocolate but ate 15 graham crackers, a bowl of cereal, and an apple—and then ate the chocolate anyway."

Her advice: Indulge in a reasonable portion of the food you crave, unless it's a trigger food that may lead you into a binge. (In that case, proceed to Commandment #6.)

There's a correct way to feed your craving, too, adds Dr. Turner. Put one serving of the food you crave in a dish or a bowl, then put the package away. *Then* eat. "Don't read, don't talk on the phone, don't watch TV," she says. "Focus entirely on the food. Concentrate on how good it is. And when you're finished, you're finished."

Commandment #6:
Thou Shalt Use the Five Ds

This is the most difficult of all the commandments because it asks you to use your brains when you're staring down at the unopened bag of cookies. When your very soul cries out for sugar or grease. But use your gray matter you must.

"When you binge, you stop thinking. Your brain goes AWOL," says Dr. Musante. "The Five Ds give you the chance to turn your brain back on and think through your

How Many Calories Make a Binge?

In studying the eating patterns of 51 female binge eaters, researchers at the Ohio State University College of Nursing in Columbus found that the women ate an average of 1,809 calories on the days they didn't binge. On the days they let loose, they ate an average of 2,707 calories—a 66 percent increase.

impulse to eat." When you are about to embark on a binge (or are already started on one), follow these steps.

Determine what's going on. Ask yourself, "Why do I want to eat so badly right now?"

Delay your response by figuring out what's driving your urge to eat. Are you famished because you skipped a meal? Angry? Bored? Lonely? You might feel that once you've hit this point, there's nothing on God's green earth that can step between you and your jumbo bag of chocolate candies. And that may be true, says Dr. Musante. "But do you have to eat them at this moment? In the next 60 seconds? You can eat them 5 minutes from now, 10 minutes from now, or an hour from now." The longer you stall, the higher the likelihood that the craving will pass.

Distract yourself for at least 10 minutes. If you're at home, take a shower or give yourself a manicure. (It's hard to binge when your nails are wet.) If you're at work, take a walk around your building, visit a colleague, or freshen up in the ladies' room.

Distance yourself from temptation. If you're at home, throw your binge food down the garbage disposal or bury it in the trash so you can't fish it out again. Leave the house if you have to. If you're out to dinner, ask the waiter to immediately wrap up half of the lumberjack-size entrée he's just set in front of you. If you go to the movies, arrive just before show time, so there's no time to hit the concession stand.

Decide how you'll handle the situation. Will you stop—or continue? "Some women decide to keep eating," says Kern. "But they do so consciously. They know what they're doing, understand why, realize the consequences, and choose to proceed. They're exercising the power of choice, which is more advanced behavior."

Commandment #7:
Thou Shalt Freeze the Moment

On TV, when a policeman yells "Freeze!" the bad guy usually does. What if you could yell "Freeze!" at the start of a binge—or even midway through?

The High Price of Bingeing

Compulsive overeating isn't just unhealthy. Here's the dollar cost of some typical pig-out portions.

> One (10.5-ounce) package of corn chips: $2.19
> One (8.5-ounce) container of dip: $2.99
> One (17-ounce) package of M&Ms: $3.29
> One (1-pound, 2-ounce) bag of chocolate chip
>   cookies: $3.19
> Two pints of gourmet ice cream: $6.98
> One frozen pizza: $5.99
> **Total: $24.63**

The upshot? If you normally binge on foods like these twice a month, learning to resist temptation could save nearly $600 a year!

You can, with a simple technique called freezing the moment, says Dr. Musante. In this technique, you stop in your tracks—perhaps with a cookie halfway to your mouth or in the act of cutting yourself a fourth brownie.

Dr. Musante tells his clients to remember a scene from one of those old *Star Trek* episodes in which the characters are frozen in time and space. "When you freeze the moment, you have the opportunity to come to your senses."

Even if you don't stop eating, freezing the moment will at least give you the opportunity to control how much you eat. For example, instead of polishing off the entire pint of gourmet ice cream, measure out ½ cup, put it in a bowl, and put the carton away. Or measure out one serving (1 ounce) of chips into a bowl and seal the bag.

Freezing the moment also reminds you that you're in control, says Kern. "If you've had two cookies and not a third, you restore your sense of control," he says. "And instead of feeling bad that you had two, you can feel good that the lapse didn't become a *collapse*."

Commandment #8:
Thou Shalt Make Emergency Stops

When you're on the road and you blow a tire, you're supposed to stay calm and pull over to the side of the road. That's exactly what you need to do, metaphorically speaking, after you overeat.

"After a binge, women inevitably feel incredible anxiety and guilt, which can send them further out of control," says Kern. So in the first minutes after a binge, counter these awful feelings. On paper, reconstruct the entire episode. Pinpoint the circumstances that led to the binge and the strategies you might have tried to halt it at any point along the way.

The very act of thinking and writing may calm you, making you more receptive to what went wrong, says

Kern. Which makes it easier to devise strategies that will help you avoid those circumstances next time. "If you learn something, then you've fallen forward rather than backward."

15 By-the-Mouthful Munchies

You want snacks. Lots of snacks. Big, whopping handfuls of snacks. When you reach for the treats below, you get quantity as well as quality. The beautiful part is that each contains no more than 250 calories and less than 10 grams of fat. To avoid too much of a good thing, indulge no more than once a week.

- 80 baked pita puffs
- 68 Sunshine Krispy soup and oyster crackers
- 65 pretzel sticks dipped in 2 tablespoons of fat-free hot fudge topping
- 43 Ritz Air Crisps (sour cream and onion flavor)
- 40 bite-size baked Tostitos, plus salsa
- 30 Orville Redenbacher's Peanut Caramel Crunch low-fat mini popcorn cakes
- 30 baby carrots with ½ cup of low-fat dip
- 11 cups of Orville Redenbacher's Natural Light popcorn
- 3 cherry Fruit-a-Freeze bars
- 2 boxes (3 ounces each) of MicroMagic low-fat french fries
- 2 snack-size bags of Baked Lays potato chips
- 2 cups of Quaker Crunchy Corn Bran
- 1 Veggie Delite sub (6-inch) from Subway
- 1 box of Nabisco Barnum's Animals crackers
- 1 baked apple, drizzled with 1 tablespoon of caramel sundae topping and sprinkled with cinnamon

Commandment #9:
Thou Shalt Not Beat Thyself Up

To bounce back from a binge, you must forgive yourself, says Dr. Musante. That means you must silence the punishing voice in your head that says you're a glutton with no willpower.

Just as jelly beans are empty calories, shame and guilt are empty emotions. "They teach us nothing," says Dr. Musante. In fact, they may actually trigger another binge. When you beat yourself up, you're more likely to turn to snack cakes to soothe yourself, says Dr. Musante. Or to starve yourself the next day, leaving yourself vulnerable to another pig-out.

When that nasty chorus in your head starts to sing, silently shout, "STOP!" says Dr. Musante. (Or shout it out loud, if you're alone.) Then replace the negative message with a positive one, for example: "Yes, I slipped. I don't feel good about it, but I don't have to beat myself up either. I hereby forgive myself. And I'll do better tomorrow."

Commandment # 10:
Thou Shalt Get Back in the Game

No matter what time of day your binge occurs and no matter how dispirited you feel, eat your next scheduled meal, advises Kern. When you immediately resume your normal eating pattern, you help fight off those "What does it matter? I've blown it so I may as well keep eating" blues.

Say you overate—big time—at lunch. "When dinnertime rolls around, simply eat the meal you'd planned to eat. It's a way to tell yourself that you're back in the game, so to speak, says Kern. And that you've begun to restore control to the person to whom it rightfully belongs—you."

The Seventh Key: Prepare for Sticky Situations

Think of your diet as a cross-country road trip. Your goal is to get from New York to Los Angeles without breaking down, getting lost, or colliding with someone or something.

To do that, you need to learn to read the danger signs, avoid the slippery slopes, and navigate the detours with ease and panache. That takes know-how, practice, and skill.

Here, then, is your map to reach dietary success.

Navigating the Salad Bar

Don't let the "S" word fool you: The average salad bar plate can pack more than 1,000 calories—more than a deluxe burger, fries, and a shake. In fact, in one study researchers found that 60 to 70 percent of the calories in a salad bar salad came from fat.

Here's how to avoid salad bar "potholes."

Take a smaller plate. Fill your dish rim to rim—but not sky high.

Disqualify fried foods and confections. This is a salad bar. Eat salad. Pass up anything batter-fried, be it chicken or zucchini. Go easy on ice cream or pudding.

Minimize the oil slick. While you may use fat-free mayo at home, salad bar salads do not. So go easy on the macaroni salad, coleslaw, and potato salad—or skip it entirely.

Pile up the veggies, beans, and fruit. They're loaded with vitamins, minerals, and fiber—with little or no fat. For more nutrients, pick dark leafy greens instead of iceberg lettuce. One cup of spinach has five times the calcium, twice the fiber, and several thousand times the vitamin A that the same amount of iceberg lettuce has.

Slim down the dressings. Two tablespoons of a traditional dressing adds about 150 calories to an otherwise low-fat plate. Splash on some balsamic vinegar and just a drizzle of olive oil instead. You'll get the flavor plus a bonus: The olive oil helps you absorb nutrient-rich carotenoids from the vegetables.

Slash the toppings. We're talking Chinese noodles and croutons. An ounce of croutons (½ cup), for instance, packs 65 calories and 2½ grams of fat.

Cruising the Buffet Table

Like a scenic mountaintop vista, buffet tables can be overwhelming. Only you can touch, smell, and taste this scenic wonder. But an expedition through an all-you-can-eat buffet isn't all that different from a trek across the Rockies. Just plan ahead and take it slow.

Map out your route. Survey each part of the buffet table—salads, soups, entrées, side dishes, breads, and desserts—before putting any food on your plate. Decide what you absolutely must have, then take it after thoughtful consideration.

Focus on getting your nutrition's worth, not your money's worth. Opt for steamed or grilled vegetables instead of those swimming in butter or cream sauce; fresh fruit versus pie topped with whipped cream; broiled poultry or fish rather than fried; and lean roasted meats. Flavor veggies and even bread with just a drizzle of olive oil, if anything. Use a splash of soy sauce for roasted meats, if needed, instead of gravy.

Take a one-way trip. Sit at a table on the other side of the room from the buffet so you won't be tempted by its aromas. Otherwise, it's just too easy to make a return trip.

Slow down. It takes about 20 minutes for your stomach to tell your brain that you're full. So put your fork down each time you try a different food.

Take it natural. Choose foods that are prepared simply: steamed shrimp, carved turkey breast, cherry tomatoes. If it's sitting in sauce or hidden under breading, go easy or skip it.

Chocolate Speed Bumps

Chocolate is a major treat for many women, and it's not hard to understand why. Nothing quite equals chocolate for flavor, creaminess, and pure indulgence. In fact, researchers now admit that a psychological chocolate craving does exist. So although we wouldn't recommend anything called the chocolate diet, we still think the luscious flavor can have a place in a woman's life. Go easy, though, because chocolate candy is loaded with calories and fat.

Consider cocoa. One ounce of cocoa powder has about 100 calories and 0.5 gram of fat, compared with 190 calories and 16 grams of fat in a 1-ounce chunk of unsweetened chocolate. Try substituting cocoa powder in baking recipes and puddings. You can even puree it

The Perfect Chocolate Treat

These fudgy squares can stop a chocolate craving cold. We lowered the fat by using cocoa powder instead of baking chocolate and replacing some of the butter with applesauce. As a result, compared with traditional walnut brownies, this recipe has about half the fat and twice the fiber. And because these brownies are dense, just one may be enough to get that yen for chocolate under control.

Nutty Brownies

  2 tablespoons melted butter
  ⅓ cup unsweetened applesauce
  ¾ cup sugar
  ½ cup unsweetened cocoa powder
  1 egg or ¼ cup fat-free liquid egg substitute
  1 teaspoon vanilla extract
  ½ cup whole wheat flour
  ⅓ cup finely chopped walnuts
     Confectioners' sugar (optional)

Preheat the oven to 350°F. Coat an 8″ × 8″ glass baking dish with cooking spray.

In a large bowl, stir together the butter and applesauce. One at a time, stir in the sugar, cocoa powder, egg or egg substitute, vanilla, flour, and walnuts until well-mixed. Spread the batter in the prepared pan.

Bake for 25 minutes, or until the sides begin to pull away from the pan. Cool in the pan on a wire rack. Cut into squares and sprinkle with the confectioners' sugar, if using.

Makes 16

Per brownie: 88 calories, 2 g protein, 14 g carbohydrates, 4 g fat, 17 mg cholesterol, 1 g dietary fiber, 21 mg sodium

with a few strawberries, fat-free milk, and ice for a low-fat smoothie.

Keep it small. Satisfy your craving with a small handful of chocolate chips, a miniature chocolate bar, or just two or three chocolate kisses. Always serve them on a plate or a napkin and put the rest away.

Go for the best. Buy the very best chocolate you can, then freeze it. When the craving hits, pop one piece into your mouth and see how much longer the lusciousness lingers. For fewer calories, choose chocolate-dipped fruit instead of chocolate fudge, chocolate angel food cake instead of devil's food cake with icing, and low-fat chocolate milk instead of a chocolate milkshake.

Cocktail Party Patrol

You're all dressed up, feeling beautiful, and networking your brains out when you realize that every other time you open your mouth it's not words going out but hors d'oeuvres going in. To eat (and drink) smarter on the cocktail party–reception–company shindig circuit, try these tips.

Water down the drinks. Just two glasses of wine or spiked punch, two mixed drinks, or two beers, and you've already downed more calories than a half-hour walk later can use up. Not to mention that the more you drink, the less willpower you may have for avoiding the buffet table. But holding a drink isn't all bad. After all, it keeps one hand away from the chicken croquettes and baked Brie.

- Drink a glass of water before each alcoholic beverage; you can even fill your empty beer bottle with water.
- Cut your wine with seltzer water and your mixed drinks with extra mixer.
- Load up your glass with ice before pouring anything into it.

- Make your own drinks in order to control the alcohol.
- Volunteer to drive. Then drink club soda or diet cola with no apologies.

Eat something beforehand. Have a bowl of soup or a piece of fruit before you arrive, so you're not facing temptation on an empty stomach. When the hors d'oeuvres make the rounds, graze selectively. Take one bite of whatever you want. Then discreetly discard your plate, pick up a clean one, and fill it with raw vegetables, steamed potstickers (small Chinese dumplings), and shrimp. (Be aware, though, that if the dumplings seem browned, they were probably pan-fried in small amounts of peanut oil.)

Pick the right hors d'oeuvres. This means making a wide turn around the Buffalo wings (200 calories and 15 grams of fat per one fried wing) and heading over to the vegetable lane. Watch out! You nearly got sideswiped by the onion dip (50 calories and 4 grams of fat per 2 tablespoons). Park yourself over by the steamed shrimp (10 calories and no fat per shrimp) and sushi (71 calories with 1 gram of fat per piece), and you can even pop a bacon-wrapped scallop in your mouth if the bacon just wraps around once (39 calories with 2 grams of fat).

Stay active. There's plenty to do besides eat and drink. Dance, take photos, admire the artwork and the view, or help your hostess serve.

The Holiday Slide

So you're driving along, doing just fine on your new eating plan—note that it's a plan, not a diet—when suddenly the weather cools and the leaves change color. In stores everywhere, Halloween candy has replaced summer lawn chairs. In back, they're unpacking Christmas ornaments.

Caution: detour ahead. For the next few months, you may find yourself swerving to avoid rich holiday cookies, trying not to get hit with fat-laden appetizers, and pushing through a blinding storm of baking, parties, and other temptations.

Tame the cookie monster. We know. What's Christmas without Christmas cookies? All 12 varieties, 36 dozen of them. The problem is that when you go to pack them into gift tins, you may have only half that number left. The rest may be providing some winter warmth around your hips. So try this.

Satisfying Low-Fat Cookies

Keep a batch of these little "snowballs" on hand for when your sweet tooth demands attention. Since they're made with egg whites—and little else—they're very low in fat. And what fat they do contain comes from the almonds and is the cholesterol-lowering, monounsaturated kind.

Toasted-Almond Kisses

    4   large egg whites, at room temperature
    ⅛   teaspoon salt
    ¾   cup confectioners' sugar
    ½   cup granulated sugar
    ¾   teaspoon vanilla extract
    ¼   teaspoon almond extract
    ½   cup toasted and very finely chopped blanched
        almonds

Preheat the oven to 250°F. Line two baking sheets with parchment paper.

Place the egg whites and salt in a large bowl. Beat with an electric mixer on low speed until foamy.

- Use applesauce, mashed bananas, or pureed fruit for half the fat in cookie recipes.
- Toast nuts to bring out the full flavor, then use only half the amount called for.
- Cut calories per cookie by making cookies smaller.
- Try gingersnaps instead of chocolate chip cookies, or oatmeal cookies instead of peanut butter cookies.
- Schedule your holiday baking right after dinner, when you're full. Then package the cookies into tins the minute they're cool, seal them with brightly colored plastic wrap, and store them upstairs in a cool, dry, out-of-the-way place until it's time to serve or deliver them.

In a small bowl, combine the confectioners' sugar and granulated sugar. Gradually add 1 tablespoon at a time to the egg whites, beating well after each addition, until the whites are stiff and shiny. Beat in the vanilla and almond extract. Gently fold in the almonds.

Drop heaping teaspoonfuls of the batter, 1" apart, onto the baking sheets.

Bake for 35 minutes, switching the position of the sheets halfway through. Turn off the oven and let the cookies stay in the oven for 30 minutes longer.

Let cool on a wire rack. Peel the cookies from the paper and store in an airtight container.

Makes 72
Per cookie: 16 calories, 0 g protein, 3 g carbohydrates, 0.5 g fat, 0 mg cholesterol, 0 g dietary fiber, 4 mg sodium

Note: It's best to bake meringue cookies on a cool, dry day or they will be too sticky.

- Buy, don't bake. A great idea if you really don't enjoy baking but need the cookies as gifts or for school parties. Just wait until the day you need them to buy the cookies, so you're less likely to raid them.

Survive the holiday dinner calorie pileup. Why do all of our celebrations revolve around at least one really big, no-holds-barred dinner? There's turkey at Thanksgiving, fried potato pancakes at Hanukkah, stuffed goose at Christmas, baked ham at Easter. . . . It takes a day or more to prepare the meal, all of 10 minutes to demolish it—and the rest of the month to work it off.

True, Christmas (and Thanksgiving, Easter, the Fourth of July, your birthday, and your husband's birthday) comes only once a year. Add your niece's wedding, your nephew's graduation, ad infinitum, and celebrating soon becomes a way of life. To avoid too many just-this-once pounds:

- Take a tablespoon-size serving of each dish. By the time you eat it all, chances are you'll be satisfied.
- Discard the turkey skin. You'll save 140 calories per drumstick.
- Skip the butter for the rolls or use one pat, not two— and say so long to 35 calories that you'll never miss.

Caesar Salad: Dinner Disaster

A Caesar side salad may have only 210 calories, but it has 17 grams of fat—mainly from the anchovies, egg, oil, and cheese in the dressing. Your best bet is to get the salad without the dressing or try the romaine lettuce with oil and vinegar instead. If neither option appeals to you, at least try to get the dressing on the side so you can control how much you eat.

- Choose cranberry sauce (¼ cup has 110 calories and almost no fat) instead of gravy.
- Have cookies or dessert, but not both.
- Eat just a sliver of pie, not a whole slice.
- Stick to your regular schedule. Just because dinner is being served at 3:00 P.M. doesn't mean you should skip lunch. So have a light lunch at noon; then you won't be starving when dinner is served.
- Make an after-meal walk part of the holiday tradition.

Weekend Blowouts

Your weight-control strategies may stay on track during the routine of the workday, but let the weekend hit and all bets are off. It's like hitting the road in your father's car just after getting your driver's license for the first time. Here's how to avoid a crash.

Get out of the house. Get away from the refrigerator. Try hiking, biking, walking, or gardening. In bad weather, walk at the mall (just leave your wallet locked in the glove compartment so that you're not tempted by the cinnamon buns).

Watch out for festival food. By all means, take in craft fairs, art walks, antique shows, or jazz fests. But watch those food stands: If sausage sandwiches, cheese fries, and fried crab cakes leave your hands greasy, think of what eating too many can do to your waistline and arteries. Still, sampling food is part of the experience. Here are the alternatives.

- Stroll ahead and scout out all of your options. Opt for healthier fare (yes, it does exist), like a grilled turkey leg or a fruit smoothie.
- Carry a couple of dollars and a credit card with you. Many food vendors won't take plastic, so you're limiting the temptation.

Stroganoff That's Good for You

This notorious Russian fat trap gets a slimming makeover thanks to lower-fat yogurt and sour cream. The shiitake mushrooms lend more than just meaty taste and texture to this tater topper—studies show that they contain a variety of cancer-preventing compounds.

Baked Potatoes with Mushroom Stroganoff

    4 medium baking potatoes
    1 small onion, finely chopped
    1 tablespoon canola oil
    8 ounces shiitake mushrooms, thinly sliced
    ¼ teaspoon dried thyme
    ¼ teaspoon salt
    ¼ teaspoon ground black pepper
    2 tablespoons balsamic vinegar
    1 cup low-fat plain yogurt
    ½ cup reduced-fat sour cream

Skip the Sunday brunch. It's very tempting to grab the newspaper and head out for a "real" (that is, diner) breakfast when you don't have to report to the office. But figure that two slices of bacon, two fried eggs, and two pieces of buttered toast mean nearly 500 calories and 33 grams of fat. Instead, treat yourself to a special breakfast and the Sunday paper but keep it healthy, with a cup of egg substitute, one slice of toast spread with 1 tablespoon of jam instead of butter, and one slice of Canadian bacon. This totals 295 calories, with about 6 grams of fat.

Movie Minefields

A few years ago, a consumer watchdog group reported that movie theater popcorn is swimming in saturated fat. A

Preheat the oven to 400°F. Place the potatoes on a baking sheet and bake for 1 hour (or pierce them several times with a fork and microwave on high for 15 minutes).

In a large nonstick skillet over medium heat, cook the onion in the oil for 3 minutes. Add the mushrooms, thyme, salt, and pepper. Cook for 5 minutes. Stir in the vinegar and cook for 1 minute, or until the liquid evaporates.

In a small saucepan, whisk together the yogurt and sour cream. Stir over low heat for 5 minutes, or until warm. (Do not allow the mixture to get too hot or it will separate.)

Split the baked potatoes. Top with the yogurt mixture and the mushrooms.

Makes 4 servings

Per serving: 250 calories, 9 g protein, 38 g carbohydrates, 8 g fat, 4 mg cholesterol, 4 g dietary fiber, 209 mg sodium

large popcorn cooked in coconut oil with butter topping has about 80 grams of fat, more than 50 of them saturated. That's almost 3 days' worth of the recommended limit for this artery-clogging saturated fat, or what you'd get from six McDonald's Big Macs.

Sitting in a movie without a box of popcorn or a candy bar is like hitting the beach without shaving your legs first. You just can't do it. So instead:

Bring your own. Three-and-a-half cups of air-popped popcorn has about 110 calories; the same amount of theater popcorn has as much as 301 calories—and you know you aren't going to stop at 3½ cups. Even a kid-size order in the theater has twice that much.

Pick Jujubes. They'll take you so long to chew, the closing credits will be rolling before you finish the box.

And at 120 calories for 54 pieces (and no fat), you won't be blowing your entire diet.

Mr. Potato Head at the Wheel

You say tomato, he says french fries. You say veggie burger, he says New York strip steak. Even if you're married to a meat-and-potatoes guy who eschews "diet" food, you can plan meals that make everyone happy.

Go for the grill. He can have his meat, and you can have grilled vegetables or fish or chicken, without dirtying another dish.

Build a better burger. Add nutrients by jazzing up burgers. Start with lean meat. Try ground turkey or chicken breast, or even vegetable or salmon patties. Flavor them with great herbs like fresh dill, basil, or oregano. Use chutneys, horseradish, or gourmet mustards instead of high-fat mayo. Layer the burgers with tomato and onion slices, grilled peppers and mushrooms, or spinach leaves and pineapple slices. Also, exchange plain white-bread buns for whole wheat bread for more fiber.

Challenge him to a duel. A nutritional duel, that is. If you're trying to lose weight, chances are he could lose a few pounds, too. See who can lose 4 to 5 pounds within a month. Or see who can actually get those six to nine servings of fruits and vegetables and 30 grams of fiber a day. The loser has to do the laundry—and put it away—for the next month.

Picky Kids in Tow

How many times have you felt so proud of yourself for cooking a healthful, nutritious meal, only to have your children react as if you'd just handed them a summer

Slimming Macaroni and Cheese

There's no baking needed for this fast stovetop recipe. But what really makes this dish special is the flavor boost it gets from horseradish and tomato paste, both fat-free and low-cal.

Quick Pasta and Cheese

12	ounces elbow macaroni or medium shells
1	tablespoon butter
2	tablespoons all-purpose flour
2	cups 1% milk
2	tablespoons tomato paste
2	teaspoons Dijon mustard
2	teaspoons prepared horseradish
¾	teaspoon salt
1½	cups shredded sharp Cheddar cheese

In a large pot of boiling water, cook the pasta according to the package directions. Drain and return to the pan.

In a medium saucepan, melt the butter over medium heat. Whisk in the flour and cook, stirring, for 2 minutes. Slowly whisk in the milk and cook, stirring, for 5 minutes, or until the sauce begins to thicken. Whisk in the tomato paste, mustard, horseradish, and salt. Add the cheese and stir for 1 minute, or just until melted.

Pour the cheese mixture over the pasta. Stir over medium heat for 1 minute, or until the pasta is hot.

Makes 6 cups
Per cup: 406 calories, 20 g protein, 51 g carbohydrates, 12.5 g fat, 38 mg cholesterol, 2 g dietary fiber, 691 mg sodium

reading list? It's enough to make you buy stock in frozen chicken nuggets.

But the munchkins need a healthful diet as much as you do. Here are some ways to get your kids to eat the nutritious meals you cook without bringing child protective services to your door.

Let picky kids pick. Give them choices: Chicken or fish? Broccoli or carrots? Brown rice or polenta? But always keep the choices to two, and keep both equally healthful. You're giving your child a sense of control—without giving up smart eating yourself.

Let 'em help. Yeah, this might be asking for trouble, but it's amazing how much more delectable that swordfish looks to your 7-year-old when he's the one who got to sprinkle on the soy sauce and chopped ginger.

Sneak in the healthful food. If macaroni and cheese is all she'll eat, mix in some peas or carrots, some tuna or chicken. Instead of fried chicken nuggets, make your own and bake them. Use prepared pizza shells and load the pie with vegetables instead of pepperoni and cheese. If your child is a peanut butter lover, try stuffing celery with peanut butter or make a peanut butter sauce to go with a stir-fry.

Build your own. With these dinners, kids will be so busy creating, they won't have time to notice all the—*gasp!*—healthful ingredients.

- Build-your-own-pita-pockets night. Put out whole wheat pita bread sliced in half; small pieces of sliced turkey breast or low-fat cheese; and veggies including lettuce, sliced tomatoes, sliced onions, cucumbers, sprouts, or whatever else you like.
- Build-your-own-burrito night. Put out cooked ground turkey, cooked kidney or black beans, hot sauce, black olives, rice, torn lettuce, diced tomatoes, and warmed flour tortillas.

- Build-your-own-baked-potato night. Put out grated Parmesan cheese, fat-free plain yogurt flavored with curry or dill, ratatouille, cooked peas, salsa, steamed broccoli, and shredded low-fat Cheddar cheese.

Stick to your guns. Missing a meal won't hurt them. If they continually refuse to eat what you've fixed, then just set the rule: This is dinner. Eat it or don't, but the kitchen is now closed. You'll be amazed at how quickly they begin eating what you serve.

Office Oil Slicks

"Cake in the break room" flashes the e-mail. Before you know it, two pieces have disappeared into your mouth. Then there's the jar of chocolate candies on your boss's desk. Ever wonder why she has to refill it after every meeting with you?

And let's not even go to the snack machine. Did you know that a daily bag of 1 ounce of chips (calorie content: 150) adds up to an extra 750 calories a week? That could explain the extra pound a month you've been mysteriously accumulating.

Saunter, don't stuff. Stressed by work? Take a walk—and we don't mean to the cafeteria. If the weather won't allow stepping outside, walk the halls or up and down the stairs. Walk on a different floor where no one knows you. And don't feel guilty: Everyone is entitled to a break once in a while.

Join in—on your terms. Fit your coworkers' treats, such as a muffin or cookies, into your day's meal plan. Take one to enjoy later with lunch, rather than add that muffin as a second dessert. If it's a midafternoon pick-me-up, take the treat home for an after-dinner dessert. When it's your turn to supply the munchies, set the standard with exotic fruits, whole-grain bagels, or baby vegetables.

What's Wrong with Fried Fish

Baked, broiled, steamed, or grilled fish is a great choice. But fast-food restaurants typically offer fried-fish sandwiches—with plenty of tartar sauce—at 430 calories apiece. You're better off ordering a grilled chicken breast sandwich, at 310 calories, or even a small burger, at 275 calories.

Stick with water. While everyone is standing around the break room, nibbling cake, keep your hands and mouth busy with a bottle of water. After all, you need at least 9 cups of fluid daily. As a bonus, water won't leave a sticky mess on your computer keyboard.

Road Trip

It feels like you've been on this interstate for days. Everything looks the same—billboards, road signs, monster trucks. Then you see it: a rest stop ahead, complete with kiosks selling cinnamon buns. Watch it. If you're not careful, you could actually end this car trip weighing more than when you began since 1 hour of driving uses only about 110 calories and a Cinnabon contains 670 calories and 34 grams of fat (14 of them saturated).

There are alternatives.

Get off the main road. Instead of the ubiquitous burger and pizza chains lining interstate highways, pull onto a secondary road and look for family-style restaurants that offer more variety and other options, including grilled foods, fish that's not battered and fried, vegetables, and local specialties (unless it's chicken-fried steak).

Have a picnic. Stop at a grocery store or roadside stand and buy an instant picnic: lean deli meat, cheese, crusty whole-grain bread, fresh fruit, cartons of yogurt, raw veggies, juice, and bottled water. Keep paper plates, napkins, and a few utensils in the car and find a picturesque (or at least quiet) spot to enjoy. Even that rest stop usually has picnic benches. Take a quick walk before getting back in the car.

Shop for the car. If you're like most women, you probably spend more time in your car than you do in your kitchen. So keep it stocked with long-lasting, healthful snacks like crackers, cereal bars, juice boxes, dried fruit, nuts, pretzels, rice cakes, whole wheat crackers, and bottled water. You may not necessarily save a huge number of calories. But your meal or snack will consist of nutritious, lower-fat foods.

Excess Vacation Baggage

Just because you're leaving behind the computer, e-mail, cell phone, and deadlines doesn't mean that you should leave behind your healthy eating plan. After all, an extra 5 pounds wasn't exactly the souvenir you had in mind.

Pack appropriately. We're talking exercise clothes and athletic shoes. And use them at least once a day.

Make lunch your main meal. We figure you're going to be eating all your meals out, so save your main meal for lunch. Lunch portions are typically smaller than dinner and usually cost less. Take the afternoon to work off calories on a walking tour.

Eat like the natives. Especially if you're traveling overseas, you'll find that most countries have a great many more fruits and vegetables and whole grains served with meals. Take advantage of it.

Choose the right vacation. A spa, for instance, typically features meals and snacks consisting of fruits, vegetables, whole-grain foods, low-fat dairy foods, and lean meat, poultry, and fish. Or try an adventure vacation like skiing, visiting a dude ranch, hiking, or taking a bike tour. You'll be burning up so many calories that how much you eat probably won't be an issue.

Missing the Exit for Breakfast

When *Prevention* magazine asked women about their fantasy foods, high-fat breakfast foods like doughnuts and cinnamon buns made the top 10. Yet women are notorious breakfast skippers. We're either too busy, not hungry, or apt to save the calories for later.

Big mistake. Studies show that thin people tend to eat breakfast, while overweight people tend to skip it. They just make up for it later by overeating or making poor food choices. Here's how to eat a better breakfast, quickly and painlessly.

Drink your breakfast. Fruit smoothies are nutritious, quick, and portable. Slug yours down in the car on the way to work. Just puree fruit (peaches, bananas, kiwifruit, melon, berries, or even applesauce), fat-free yogurt, and ice into a thick, refreshing drink. Sprinkle some wheat germ, wheat bran, or instant oatmeal on top for a nutritional boost. This first-thing-in-the-morning powerhouse breakfast provides nutrients, including calcium, not to mention that it's low in fat.

Skip it now, eat it later. When mornings are too hectic or you just can't stomach food first thing, plan ahead. Tuck some fruit, a bagel, cheese and crackers, or a muffin into a bag. Stock your office refrigerator with cartons of yogurt and fat-free milk, and an empty file drawer with single-serving sizes of high-fiber cereal.

Is a Bagel Better Than a Doughnut?

If you're slathering a super-size bagel with cream cheese, you might as well have the doughnut. Two tablespoons of regular cream cheese adds 100 calories and 10 grams of fat to that 195-calorie, practically fat-free bagel, for a total of 295 calories. The doughnut isn't much different, supplying about 245 calories and 15 grams of fat.

Try half a bagel with fat-free cream cheese, which has just 32 calories and barely 1 gram of fat in 2 tablespoons.

Jump-start your morning the night before. Fill your cereal bowl, slice fruit, hard-cook an egg, reconstitute juice, set the timer so your bread machine bakes while you sleep, or assemble a breakfast sandwich (perhaps raisin bread, lean ham, and cheese)—wrap it up and have it waiting in the fridge.

Forget dessert for breakfast. It's tempting, what with sweet muffins, pastries, and doughnuts all considered breakfast foods. But if you grab a large almond croissant, you'll get more fat and calories than in two Dove Bars.

Watch out for the fast-food breakfast. McDonald's bagel sandwiches have at least double the fat and the calories of the 290-calorie Egg McMuffin.

Try these great grab-and-go breakfasts.

- Spread 2 tablespoons of hummus (chickpea spread) on half a pumpernickel bagel.
- Stuff half a whole wheat pita with ½ cup of 1% cottage cheese and sliced peaches, pears, or banana.
- Roll up a tortilla with scrambled egg substitute and salsa.

Lunch on the Lam

In between running errands to the dry cleaner, bank, and drugstore, you realize you're starving. Small wonder. It is, after all, your *lunch* hour. So you see a burger haven and hit the blinker.

Go beyond burgers and fries. Search for the unique. A box of sushi from the ready-to-eat grocery section. A turkey sub from Subway. A bagel sandwich with low-fat fillings.

If you can't get out of your car and fast food is the only thing for miles, then order smart. A deluxe bacon cheeseburger, large fries, and a 12-ounce soft drink can weigh in at a whopping 1,185 calories and 52 grams of fat. A plain hamburger and a small salad with fat-free dressing have only 345 calories with 9 grams of fat. A grilled chicken sandwich with no sauce has about 300 calories with 5 grams of fat. Add a carton of low-fat milk; you need the calcium.

Eating at Your Desk

If you're not out running errands during lunch, you're probably wolfing it down at your desk between phone calls and e-mails. We call this mindless eating. Taste anything? Feel anything? A better strategy is to eat deliberately. Here's how.

Don't Eat and Drive

Half of all auto accidents occur because the driver isn't paying attention, according to the National Highway Traffic Safety Administration. If you have to run those errands at lunch, don't try to eat on the run. Instead, pack a sandwich and fruit and find 5 minutes at a picnic table somewhere, or even eat in your car at a park.

Order smart to eat in. Keep a file of interesting take-out menus—with their nutrition facts, if possible—so your choices stretch beyond burgers and fries or a pale vending machine sandwich of cold cuts and white bread.

Prepare once, eat twice. You're cooking healthy for dinner these days, so double the recipe, then pack a portion in a container for lunch the next day.

Grocery shop for the office. Chances are there's a refrigerator somewhere in your building and a few inches of space in a desk drawer. Stock up on low-fat soups and bean stews, single-serving cans of tuna packed in spring water, low-fat crackers and whole wheat breads, canned fruits and unsweetened applesauce, yogurt, bananas, apples, and oranges. For impromptu lunches, keep a stack of paper plates and plastic forks, spoons, and knives in the drawer.

The Business Lunch Binge

If you're like the average woman, you eat out about four times a week, usually lunch. And if you're on an expense account, you're likely to overdo it. Unless you:

Order simply good foods. Go for something broiled or grilled, without gravies and rich sauces. See how many servings of fruits and vegetables you can get at this meal—even without the ubiquitous chicken Caesar salad.

Make it your main meal. Promise yourself that supper will be some cut-up fruit, raw veggies, yogurt, and two crackers.

Be first. Order before anyone else to avoid letting others' choices influence you.

Order extra veggies. They'll fill you up without the calories of french fries.

Maintain balance. Have one splurge per restaurant trip and then round out the meal with healthful favorites. If you have to have the fettuccine Alfredo, have a big tossed salad as an appetizer, and fruit for dessert.

Take charge. Pick the restaurant yourself, preferably one that offers healthful choices and is good about special menu requests, like no butter sauce on the fish and salad dressing served on the side.

Blinded by Night Eating

You gave the counter a final wipe, hung up the kitchen towel, and turned out the lights at 7:15 P.M. So why are you back in the kitchen 2 hours later, rooting around in the fridge like a wild boar in a patch of truffles?

Here are some ways to avoid the late-night nibbles.

Get enough during the day. Make a concerted effort to eat breakfast, a midmorning snack, a healthful lunch (not an iceberg lettuce salad), midafternoon snack, and a complete dinner (not a bowl of air-popped popcorn).

Save your dinner dessert. Is it a sweet craving? Then have dessert later. Try low-fat, low-calorie choices like fresh peaches over frozen yogurt, berries on angel food cake, apple cobbler with oatmeal crumb topping, or fresh fruit–topped custard.

Reach for fruit. This is your last chance to get the recommended minimum quota of six servings a day of fruits and vegetables for the day. Because they're high in carbohydrates, fruits leave your stomach faster than gooey, rich desserts, so you may feel more comfortable at bedtime. Another filling, healthful evening snack is a bowl of high-fiber cereal with fat-free milk.

Just do something. Walk the dog, call a friend, put a load of clothes in the washer, or light an aromatic candle and take a bubble bath. And if TV is your version of Pavlov's bell, turn it off. Break the habits that make you eat at night and you'll break the night-eating habit.

The Eighth Key: Plan for Plateaus

Many people who have tried weight-loss plans know that there are peaks and valleys to paring off pounds. At first, the weight loss can be dramatic—perhaps 2 or 3 pounds a week—then things start to slow, or stop altogether, for a time.

Nutritionists define this as a plateau. We might describe it as the special circle of hell reserved for dieters. What better words express the frustration of stepping on the scale and finding that, although you've been watching what you eat and exercising faithfully, you weigh the same amount you did last week and the week before that?

No one knows what triggers a plateau or why some people are especially vulnerable to them, says Franca Alphin, R.D., a licensed dietitian and administrative director of the Duke University Diet and Fitness Center in Durham, North Carolina. "Some people may never hit a plateau, while others may hit one 3 weeks into their program and stay there for 4 weeks," she says.

So why does the scale get stuck in the first place? There are a few possible explanations. One theory is that a plateau may be your body's way of saying, "Hey! I need time to adjust to those lost pounds."

"When you eat less and exercise more, your body's hundreds of thousands of physiological processes change somewhat," says Alphin. "A plateau may be a catch-up mechanism that allows your body to adjust to these changes." Another possible cause is water retention. "The theory is that over time, your body accumulates water, which is the end result of fat metabolism."

Or—and this is tough to admit—perhaps you've simply let your good intentions slide a bit.

Strike a Balance

The trimmer you get, the less effective your current diet and exercise program becomes—and the more likely you are to hit a plateau.

Why? Because the regimen that whittled you down from 175 to 150 pounds is unlikely to burn enough calories to get you to your goal weight of 140 pounds.

If you were 175 pounds when you started, your body burned 1,829 calories a day without exercise to maintain that weight. During exercise—for example, a daily 60-minute walk—you burned an extra 366 calories. In short, you burned 366 calories a day more than your body needed to maintain your "before" weight. Voilà!—the pounds peeled right off.

But at 150 pounds, your body requires only 1,568 calories. Further, at your new, lighter weight, the same hour-long walk burns only 312 calories. If you're still consuming 1,829 calories a day, you're not expending the number of calories necessary to drop to your goal weight of 140 pounds (1,464 calories).

"You're either consuming more calories than you did at the start of your weight-loss program or you're not exercising as much. Or possibly both," says Geralyn Coopersmith, an exercise physiologist, certified strength and conditioning specialist, and certified personal trainer at Trainer's Place in New York City. But regardless of what caused your plateau, one thing is certain: It's at this point that the tough keep going.

"Plateaus are a normal part of losing weight," says Susan Bartlett, Ph.D., assistant professor of medicine and a psychologist specializing in weight management at Johns Hopkins University School of Medicine in Baltimore. "The best thing to do is carefully evaluate whether or not you really are following your program. In most cases, there's been a slow but gradual return to old habits, and that is what is causing the plateau. If you really are doing what you need to do, the plateau is a temporary blip. Stay the course, and soon your weight loss will resume."

There are, however, a few tips and tricks you can employ to help bust a plateau, says Alphin, "assuming that your goal weight is realistic and achievable." The following two-part plan may just unstick the needle on your scale—quickly and safely.

Get Calories under Control

Whether your plateau is a normal, natural part of weight loss or the result of a few too many run-ins with your favorite treats, the answer is to burn more calories than you're taking in. Here's how to get started.

Monitor "portion drift." Many women who get tantalizingly close to their goal weights unconsciously start eating larger and larger portions, says Michelle Munyon, R.D., outpatient nutrition specialist for the Kennedy Health System, a community-based hospital system in Voorhees, New Jersey. To get back on track, arm yourself with a measuring cup and a food scale, and measure out portions every day for 1 week, she suggests. Once you've reacquainted yourself with what one serving of pasta or chicken salad actually looks like, measure or weigh your food choices 1 day a week to keep yourself honest.

Simplify portion control. Stock your freezer with frozen "light" meals. You'll know exactly how many calories you are consuming—and save yourself the hassle of measuring portions.

Eat some skinny minis. Eating mini-meals every 3 to 4 hours can help keep your blood sugar steady, which can quell hunger pangs and thereby make it easier for you to stick to your diet, says Lorna Pascal, R.D., a nutrition consultant for the Dave Winfield Nutrition Center at the Hackensack University Medical Center in New Jersey.

For example, instead of "spending" all your calories on three meals, you might eat five or six mini-meals a day—three squares plus a midmorning, midafternoon, and prime-time snack, says Pascal. Limit each mini-meal to 250 to 350 calories. For best results, include some protein. Here's an example of a day's meals.

Breakfast: ¾ cup of whole-grain cereal with half a banana, sliced, and ½ cup of fat-free milk (192 calories)

Midmorning: 1 cup of seedless grapes and a container of low-fat yogurt (257 calories)

Lunch: One small whole wheat roll, ½ cup of sliced fresh fruit (339 calories)

Midafternoon: 1 ounce of Cheddar cheese, five whole wheat crackers, one small apple (266 calories)

Dinner: 3 ounces of broiled lean meat, one small baked potato, 1 cup of steamed asparagus, one small melon wedge (345 calories)

Prime-time snack: 3 cups of air-popped popcorn flavored with Butter Buds (97 calories)

Total calories: 1,496

A Plateau or Your Perfect Weight?

Sometimes, what seems like a plateau isn't. Before you decide whether you should even bother trying to lose that last 5 or 10 pounds, consider the following questions.

Are you strength training? Then your weight may be fine where it is. Muscle gained during strength training is heavier than fat. But it's also healthier—and it looks better, too.

Where's the weight? If your extra pounds are around your middle, you might want to continue your program. Weight on the abdomen could be increasing your risk of heart disease, diabetes, and some types of cancer.

What do the numbers say? If your cholesterol, blood pressure, or blood sugar numbers are rising or high, you may want to stay with your diet. Elevated levels in any of these areas may be the first indications that your weight is affecting your health.

Are you living on planet Earth? Is it realistic to eat any less or exercise any more than you already are?

One caveat: "Women who are binge eaters or compulsive eaters are usually not good candidates for the minimeal approach because they may not be able to limit how much they eat at one sitting," says Alphin.

Redistribute your calories. Do you tend to skimp on breakfast and lunch and eat a huge dinner? Bad idea, says Alphin. You tend to burn calories consumed at night more slowly because you are not as physically active then. Instead, consume the bulk of your calories at breakfast and lunch, and eat a lighter dinner. "You're more physically active during the day, so you have higher calorie needs. You'll also burn off the bulk of those calories during the day," she says.

Eat more. If you've been following a diet of fewer than 1,200 calories a day (think of those "Lose 5 pounds in 5 days!" diets in the women's magazines), your metabolism assumes that your body is starving, says Pascal. So it starts burning calories more slowly—just what you *don't* need. Her advice is to consume an extra 100 to 200 calories a day for 1 week. It may be enough to flip off your metabolism's starvation switch.

Make like a sponge. Drink a minimum of eight 8-ounce glasses of water a day. "When you're dehydrated, your body conserves fluid," says Alphin. "Drinking more water may allow you to shed some of it."

Revamp Your Workout

Shaking up your workout may also help propel you out of a plateau. The following strategies can help you burn more calories during your workouts—and may nudge the needle on the scale southward once again.

Become a workout klutz. You've heard the expression "Work smarter, not harder." That's exactly what your muscles do when they have been performing the same workout over and over. And the more efficient your body becomes, the fewer calories you burn.

The solution? Switch to a different workout, says Coopersmith. Let's say walking is your exercise of choice. "If you start swimming, your body will be very inefficient because it will be using different muscles and movements," she says. "The good news is that inefficiency burns more calories." While the increased calorie burn amounts to only a few calories per minute, "those calories really add up during the course of a workout."

Stretch out your workout. "Another way to burn more calories is to exercise longer," says Coopersmith. She suggests extending the length of your workouts by 10 percent

You're Not Alone

In a *Prevention/NBC Today* survey, 70 percent of women reported hitting weight-loss plateaus despite having followed their diet and exercise programs to the letter.

every 2 weeks. For example, if you normally walk 30 minutes, start walking another 3 minutes. After 2 weeks, shoot for just over 36 minutes. In 3 months, you should be able to walk a whole hour.

Too busy for an hour-long workout? Break it into two 30-minute sessions. You might walk for 30 minutes at lunch and then get on the treadmill for the length of your favorite prime-time sitcom.

Lift pounds to drop pounds. When you lose extra pounds, you typically lose muscle right along with them. This loss of your body's calorie-burning machinery depresses your metabolism, so you burn fewer calories.

To lose fat without losing calorie-burning muscle, add resistance training to your workout program, recommends Melyssa St. Michael, a certified personal trainer and owner of UltraFit Human Performance, a personal training and nutrition facility in Lutherville, Maryland. For every pound of muscle you build, you burn an extra 40 to 50 calories per day.

What's more, strength training for 45 minutes at a moderate intensity also increases your resting metabolism from 25 to 30 percent for 4 hours afterward, says St. Michael, and that further increases your calorie burn.

Pump up the intensity of your workouts. Incorporating interval training (alternating short, intense bouts of exercise with slower, "recovery" phases) is another primo calorie burner, says Coopersmith.

Let's say you walk at a pace of 4 miles per hour. "To pump up the intensity, walk for 1 minute at a 4.5- to 4.8-mile-per-hour pace, and repeat this every 3 minutes," she says. "During that higher-intensity minute, you burn slightly more calories than normal." Alternate between these speeds for the entire length of your workout. If you use a treadmill or stationary bike, "try their built-in, preset interval programs," says Coopersmith.

How intense your intervals are depends on your level of fitness, she adds. If you're reasonably fit, you might want to do intervals at the highest intensity for 30 to 45 seconds. If you're working toward getting in shape, try doing intervals of moderate intensity for 1 to 3 minutes.

PART TWO

Your Natural Fat-Burning Arsenal

Natural Fat Burner #1: Food

After Susanne Holt, Ph.D., a nutrition researcher with the Commonwealth Scientific and Industrial Research Corporation in Adelaide, Australia, discovered some of the world's most satisfying edibles, she didn't leave her scientific findings locked up in a laboratory.

Instead, her "super-satisfaction foods"—from apples to fish, potatoes to whole wheat spaghetti, and beyond—have starring roles at Dr. Holt's own table when she sits down to a meal or grabs a quick afternoon snack. Thanks to her research, she is also extra-careful when the urge for classic "comfort foods" strikes because she has evidence that these tempting goodies actually fill us with calories, but they don't fill our stomachs with satisfaction.

"I'm very wary about chocolate, cakes, and ice cream," she says. "Do I really want to eat all those calories and not be satisfied? Other sweet treats—such as fruits, breakfast cereals, and low-fat yogurt—are more filling and have fewer calories."

In her research, performed at the human nutrition unit of the University of Sydney, Dr. Holt and her colleagues discovered that some surprisingly low calorie foods have significantly more power to fill you up and keep you feeling satisfied for hours than do high-calorie, high-fat treats.

Choosing more of these super satisfiers could help you eat less and burn off excess fat and weight, or maintain the healthy weight that you have already achieved—without your ever feeling hungry, according to Dr. Holt.

Maximum Pleasure, Minimum Calories

In the University of Sydney study, students ate 240-calorie portions of 38 different foods. Then they rated their feelings of hunger or fullness every 15 minutes. At the end of 2 hours came the ultimate satisfaction test: The students were turned loose at a buffet table and allowed to eat as much food as they liked while researchers noted how much they consumed.

When the crumbs settled, it was clear that the students who had eaten the most filling foods ate less food overall. The humble boiled potato, for example, emerged as a satisfaction superstar, rated seven times more filling than the same calorie portion of croissants.

Basing their ratings on a scale that assigned white bread an automatic score of 100, the researchers discovered that, calorie for calorie, cakes, doughnuts, candy bars, and ice cream were less satisfying than white bread.

Meanwhile, apples, oranges, whole wheat pasta, fish, and oatmeal were twice as satisfying. Potatoes were three times as satisfying as white bread.

What gives the super satisfiers their stomach-pleasing power, a power the researchers call satiety? "High-satiety foods were low in calories and low in fat," notes Dr. Holt. As a result, you could eat a bigger portion for the same number of calories.

Consider the potato and the croissant: 240 calories of potato weighs in at a whopping 13 ounces—nearly an en-

Super Satisfiers

Stomach growling? Here's how foods rate when it comes to satisfying hunger pangs, according to researchers at the University of Sydney in Australia. Choosing a food from the top of the list (high satiety index scores) can help fill you up with the fewest calories. For example, a plain potato is more than twice as satisfying as french fries, and 3½ times as satisfying as potato chips.

Food	Satisfaction Rating
Potatoes	323
Fish	225
Oatmeal	209
Oranges	202
Apples	197
Pasta, whole wheat	188
Beefsteak	176
Grapes	162
Popcorn, fat-free, air-popped	154
Cereal, bran	151
Cheese	146
Crackers, water	127
Cookies, crunchy	120
Bananas	118
French fries	116
Bread, white	100
Ice cream	96
Potato chips	91
Candy bars	70
Doughnuts	68
Cakes	65
Croissants	47

tire pound of food. But 240 calories of croissant weighs in at just over 2 ounces—one-sixth as much food. This difference relates to something called energy density—that is, getting a lot of nutrients combined with low amounts of calories.

Carbohydrates. The Satisfaction Specialists

Why does energy density matter? The obvious answer is that the more weight or volume of food for a given number of calories, the fuller you will feel and the less likely you will be to overeat, notes Barbara Rolls, Ph.D., professor of nutrition and director of the laboratory for the study of human ingestive behavior at Pennsylvania State University in University Park.

But beyond mere bulk, there are substances inside the super satisfiers that can keep you feeling content for hours, Dr. Holt notes. Foods like potatoes, oranges, apples, and whole grains are rich in carbohydrates, which increase blood sugar levels and stimulate receptors in your body. These in turn send a loud and clear message to brain and belly that energy stores have been replenished and satisfaction has been achieved.

And that's not all. Your stomach will digest the high-satisfaction superstars more slowly than the low-satisfaction duds, Dr. Holt says. The longer the food stays in your stomach, the longer you feel full.

What's responsible for this slow digestion? In super-satisfaction meats like lean beef and fish—cooked with little or no added fat—it's the protein, Dr. Holt says.

In fruits, vegetables, and whole grains, it's complex carbohydrates not often found in refined foods, says Paul Lachance, Ph.D., professor of food science and nutrition at Rutgers University in New Brunswick, New Jersey. "They've been shown to be more long-lasting. Digestion is slow. That's why foods like plain potatoes aren't the culprits in weight gain; a simple potato will fill you up for very few calories. In contrast, when you eat carbohydrates called simple sugars, found in refined foods like cakes and cookies, they're digested very, very quickly."

Eat-Slow Snacks

Foods that are hard to eat take longer to finish, and that gives your brain a chance to catch up with what's in your stomach, says Michelle Berry, R.D., a research nutritionist at the University of Pittsburgh and a nutrition counselor.

"It takes 20 minutes for signals of satisfaction to reach your brain. Eat slowly and you will be less likely to overeat," she says. Here are snacks that satisfy without overdoing the calories.

- Two big whole grain hard pretzels. Dip each bite into mustard or barbecue sauce.
- Five low-fat crackers topped with fat-free cream cheese and vegetables. Make up the crackers one at a time, and eat one before you make the next, Berry suggests. Doing so permits time to check for hunger and satisfaction.
- Nachos made with 15 baked tortilla chips, salsa, fat-free bean dip, and low-fat cheese.
- Make-it-yourself potato wedges instead of chips. Slice a potato into slim wedges and place on a pan spritzed with no-stick spray. Sprinkle with pepper and paprika and bake at 425°F until done (approximately 15 minutes).
- 4 cups of air-popped popcorn
- An artichoke, eaten leaf by leaf. Dip into fat-free salad dressing.
- A baked apple
- 15 frozen grapes

The fiber found in fruits, vegetables, and grains also lends a hand, keeping digestion slow and steady. The fiber also fills the stomach, Dr. Holt adds.

Slow-Motion Eating

Another big difference between super-satisfaction foods and low-satisfaction duds is ease of eating, Dr. Holt says.

"The bulkiness of the high-satisfaction foods means that it takes quite a bit of chewing before you can swallow them," she notes. This chewing gives your body and your brain more time to react to the food—which means you won't eat as many calories before you receive the "I feel full" message from your stomach.

But the low-satiety foods slip in quickly and quietly— "They melt in your mouth," Dr. Holt says. "You want to eat more."

Yet our mouths may crave low-satisfaction foods, she notes. They rule the taste buds and may even release feel-good substances in the brain that produce a feeling of happiness. "These foods increase the risk of eating a lot of calories without even realizing it," she notes. "They taste so good that you still want more, even though you've already eaten quite a lot of calories."

Choosing foods like an apple or an orange over a candy bar or a slice of cake can require restraint and patience, Dr. Holt says. "It can take effort to retrain your taste buds, but it's worthwhile. With time, you come to prefer low-fat, filling foods. You should make the changes gradually, however, and allow yourself an occasional treat."

Putting Super Satisfaction on Your Plate

Choosing the super satisfiers lets you stretch your calories while fitting in plenty of good taste and nutrition— without going hungry. Customize this strategy by switching the low-satisfaction foods that you eat most often for high-satisfaction alternatives. Here's how.

Take the gradual approach. First, tackle the highest-fat foods you eat on a regular basis, Dr. Holt says. The most important thing is to change the high-fat staples in your diet, including dairy and meat products, to leaner versions. If you tend to dine on high-fat meats, try a lower-fat alternative like skinless poultry, fish, or lower-fat beef. Also, if you snack on high-fat sweets like cakes, ice cream, or cookies, reach for fruit instead.

Choose "whole" foods. Reach for whole fruit, instead of fruit juice. Select whole grains—brown rice, whole wheat bread, whole wheat pasta—instead of foods made with refined flour. "Look for unprocessed foods, with the fiber intact," Dr. Holt suggests. In addition to keeping you full now and for hours to come, whole foods often have more nutrients than refined versions.

Reach for vegetables first. High in fiber, low in fat, and super-low in calories, vegetables have all the attributes that count in a high-satisfaction food. Try for at least three servings a day—and for extra satisfaction make each serving a full cup, suggests nutritionist Linda Gigliotti, R.D., health education coordinator for the University of California, Irvine, corporate health program and a certified diabetes expert. Add a baked potato or an ear of corn to lunch or dinner. Take a can of vegetable soup to work for lunch.

Crunch, don't sip, your juice. Naturally juicy fruits and vegetables—such as watermelon, peaches, tomatoes, and peppers—have a high water content, another attribute of high-satisfaction foods. These whole foods require more chewing and swallowing than the more processed versions. These factors slow down the rate of eating, and the whole foods take up more space in your stomach. So let crunchiness and juiciness guide you to satisfying choices.

Include some protein. Beans, lentils, and low-fat meats such as fish and poultry got high marks from eaters in Dr. Holt's satisfaction study. Including moderate amounts of lean meats at lunch and dinner can help you feel more full and give more long-term satisfaction than a salad and a piece of bread ever could, Dr. Holt says.

"Many zealous dieters who have very low fat, very high carbohydrate diets try to cut all dairy products and meats out of their diets and wonder why they still feel hungry all the time," she says. "You really need adequate, not high, amounts of low-fat protein foods in your diet to make you feel 100 percent satisfied." Consider chili made with beans and some lean ground beef, a stir-fry made with vegetables and lean

Chocolate Cures

Nutrition experts aren't sure why women love chocolate, though one theory holds that it boosts feel-good brain chemicals. Happily, there are lots of healthy ways to satisfy a chocolate urge.

- Cook-it-yourself chocolate pudding made with skim milk
- Two regular-size chocolate chip cookies (only 6 more calories than two fat-free chocolate cookies)
- Two big and crunchy chocolate wafers
- Fat-free, low-calorie hot chocolate mix
- Cocoa made with skim milk
- A snack-size candy bar
- Two individually wrapped candies—chocolate-covered cherries, peanut butter cups, chocolate mints
- Chocolate sorbet, with chocolate syrup
- One fudge pop
- Low-fat chocolate milk

meat cooked in stock instead of oil, or a curry made with chickpeas and vegetables. Or, using fat-free chicken broth, make a soup brimming with noodles, vegetables, and beans.

Fiber up. Maximize the fiber in meals and snacks to increase satisfaction, Dr. Holt suggests. Leave the skin on fruits like apples, pears, and peaches and on vegetables like eggplant, cucumbers, potatoes, and carrots—just scrub well before cooking and eating.

Think twice about reduced-fat fare. Refined low-fat foods like reduced-fat and fat-free ice cream, cookies, cakes, and candies don't have the power to fill you up.

In fact, such fare can have nearly as many calories as full-fat foods, Dr. Holt notes. Consider chocolate chip cookies: The regular cookie of one well-known brand has 53 calories, while the reduced-fat version has 50 calories. "Eating large amounts of low-fat and fat-free foods will not help people lose weight because these foods are very high in calories," she says.

Give it a little time. If you make the switch from high-fat, refined foods at meals and snacks to lower-fat, higher-fiber foods, give your taste buds about 2 weeks to adjust, Dr. Holt says. "If you stick with these foods, pretty soon you will find high-fat foods unpleasant."

Give yourself a break. Once you're eating super-satisfaction foods on a regular basis, an occasional indulgence won't threaten your waistline or your new eating habits. "A piece of cake or some chocolate once or twice a week won't hurt," Dr. Holt says.

Mini-Meals: A Small Miracle

How can something small make a big difference in whether or not you lose weight? Mini-meals make use of a primitive and powerful biological reflex, left over from our hunter-gatherer days, when food could be scarce.

When your stomach is empty for extended periods of time—say, if you eat only one meal a day—that reflex orders your metabolism to burn fewer calories. When your stomach has some food in it, that reflex tells your metabolism to speed up. So when you eat small amounts of food every 3 to 4 hours, your metabolism keeps burning extra calories—meaning that you can eat the same amount of food per day but lose more weight, says Anne Dubner, R.D., a nutrition consultant in Houston and a spokesperson for the American Dietetic Association.

Some experts theorize that mini-meals work with your stomach in another way, by keeping it the right size. When you eat a huge meal, you overfill the 3-cup capacity of your stomach. In fact, you stretch it out—and that larger stomach needs more food to feel full. So you eat more the next time. Mini-meals prevent all that.

Eating mini-meals also helps you avoid overeating, says Dubner. When you eat three (or fewer) meals a day, you get hungry between meals, she explains. You begin to think about food—a lot. And when you finally sit down to a meal, you tend to overeat. But when you eat small, frequent meals, you fill up every time you get close to a hunger pang. You never crave food. You are always satisfied, says Dubner.

Variety Is the Key

You want to continue to eat from all the food groups throughout the day: grains, fruits, vegetables, dairy products, and proteins. But you don't need to balance your intake of food groups at every meal as you did when you were eating three meals. Instead, you want to achieve balance over the course of an entire day, which means about six grains, two fruits, three vegetables, two dairy products, and two to three meat or protein products each day. (Be sure to take a calcium supplement for strong bones.)

Your Two Most Important Mini-Meals

They're an after-dinner snack and breakfast. Want to know why?

The main purpose of eating mini-meals is to keep your metabolism revved up so that you burn extra calories. But there's a time during every day when it's impossible to eat—when you're asleep. So you need a mini-meal between dinner and bedtime to keep your calorie burners stoked, says Natalie Payne, R.D., a dietitian at the Washington Cancer Institute and Washington Hospital Center in Washington, D.C. And you need to eat your breakfast mini-meal first thing in the morning.

What to eat? Payne suggests that 1 to 2 hours before bedtime you nibble on a banana, some popcorn, or a slice of whole wheat bread. In the morning, have cereal, a bagel, or half a sandwich.

But that isn't a rigid formula, says Donna Weihofen, R.D., a nutritionist at the University of Wisconsin Hospital and Clinics in Madison. You can increase or decrease servings in any category, she says—as long as you make sure to eat more grains and produce and less dairy and meat.

What's the right number of meals? It's up to you. It might be four, six, or eight. Let your body tell you what to do: Eat when you're hungry, stop when you're full, says Weihofen.

Learning to listen to your hunger might take practice; so might stopping when you're full. Here is the best advice from experts to quickly and easily adjust to mini-meals.

Keep a diary. A food diary can help you identify emotions that may trigger eating when you're not hungry, says Keith Ayoob, R.D., Ed.D., director of nutrition services at the Rose F. Kennedy Center at Albert Einstein College of Medicine of Yeshiva University in New York City. Each time you eat, write down what you ate, when you ate it, what you were doing when you ate it, and how you felt.

Make a plan. Don't wait until you're hungry to decide what to eat; hunger makes chocolate cake look like a balanced mini-meal. Plan your day's meals the night before or first thing in the morning, says Dr. Ayoob, and bring your food with you. That way, you'll have low-fat, low-calorie foods ready when the hunger hits.

Select a serving. Favor foods already portioned into individual servings, like a baked potato, a container of yogurt, or a bagel. Eating a set portion ensures that you will stop when full (or nearly full) because you will run out of food, says Michele Harvey, R.D., a diabetes educator and private nutrition consultant in Boca Raton and Delray Beach, Florida.

Slow down. Your stomach tells your brain when it's full—but it takes 20 minutes for your brain to register the message. If you eat slowly, you're more likely to realize you're full before you overeat, says Frances Oppenheimer, R.D., a dietitian at Loyola University Medical Center in Maywood, Illinois.

The best way to slow down? Have a conversation. The worst way to slow down? Watch television. People who eat while watching television tend to eat robotically, says Oppenheimer—mindlessly, quickly, and way too much.

Choose no-risk foods. As you adapt, says Dubner, choose low-calorie foods like popcorn or raw vegetables. That way, if you overeat, you'll add only a few extra calories.

Go to pieces. Mini-meals will be more satisfying if you eat them in small bites, says Dubner. So, instead of one big rice cake, have a few of the bite-size variety. Instead of eating a big pretzel, have lots of small ones. Even take a cookie, cut it into pieces, and eat each piece.

Don't tempt yourself. If you know that you have no resistance to something, stay away from it. You'd probably end up eating well beyond fullness. Choose mini-meal foods that you know you can control, says Weihofen.

Watch out for fat-free food traps. Fat-free foods won't fill you up for long. Also, many fat-free foods have lots of added sugary calories, says Weihofen, to make up for the loss of fat.

Schedule your meals. If you can't seem to master mini-meals, create an eating schedule with six meals a day, 3 hours apart, says Harvey. Once you get on a regular schedule, you'll more easily notice your body's hunger cues. For example, if you eat breakfast every morning at 7:00 A.M., your body will become hungry at that time.

Mealtime—Six Times a Day

Sometimes when people first switch to mini-meals, they find they don't have the time to prepare the food—let alone time to eat it. But eating mini-meals doesn't have to be time-consuming, says Natalie Payne, R.D., a dietitian at the Washington Cancer Institute and Washington Hospital Center in Washington, D.C. Here are some time-saving strategies.

Divide and conquer. Divide your three meals in half to create six, says Dubner. If you usually eat a bagel for breakfast, for example, eat half when you get up and the other half later. If you have a sandwich for lunch, eat the two halves at different times. That way, you won't spend any more time preparing food.

Switch meals. Consider some easy-to-prepare, easy-to-eat (but somewhat unusual) choices for your meals, says Payne. For example, make a turkey sandwich the night before, grab it from the fridge on your way out the door, and eat it for breakfast when you get to work.

Keep it cold. If you work in an office where you don't have access to a refrigerator, freeze a juice box overnight and put it in the bottom of your lunch bag the following day. The frozen juice will keep items such as yogurt and cheese cold, says Payne.

Stash some safe bets. At work, keep a desk drawer filled with canned fruit (in water or fruit juice), dried fruit, low-fat crackers, and other nonperishable convenience

Mini-Meals Aren't for Everyone

True, mini-meals are a good eating plan for people trying to lose weight.

But they don't work for everyone. Some people, for instance, have runaway appetites. Once they start eating, they keep eating until they are stuffed, says Donna Weihofen, R.D., a nutritionist at the University of Wisconsin Hospital and Clinics in Madison. Such people would be better off eating only a few times a day, she says.

Also, your lifestyle can make switching to mini-meals too difficult. For instance, if you work at a job where you cannot eat at your desk (like an assembly line) and you have only one lunch break, mini-meals may not be your best option, says Frances Oppenheimer, R.D., a dietitian at Loyola University Medical Center in Maywood, Illinois.

Give mini-meals a chance. But if you find that you can't make the switch, know that you are not a failure. And know that mini-meals are just one weight-loss option.

foods, suggests Payne. (And don't forget the can opener if your foods don't come in pop-top cans.)

Slice at night. When slicing up carrots and other raw vegetables for dinner, slice extras to munch on the next day while at work, suggests Payne.

Dinner—Your Biggest Challenge

Dinner can be the toughest time to eat a mini-meal. If you go out to eat, you're served too much food. If you eat at home, you might linger at the table with the family—and eat more than you planned. Here are some ways to think small at dinnertime.

Have an appetizer. Have a snack ready in the fridge for when you walk in the door after work, says Dubner. After you have eaten, change into comfortable clothes, take a shower, or do whatever else you do to ready yourself for an evening meal with your family. Then spend as much time at the dinner table as you like—but you won't overeat because you won't be as hungry.

Don't stay on course. Instead, switch back and forth between courses—by alternating every bite of your main dish (say chicken or pasta) with a bite of salad. If you do that, says Dubner, your food will last as long as your family's.

Fill 'er up. Before ordering dinner at a restaurant, drink a glass or two of water to quiet your appetite, says Dubner. Then take a sip of water before every bite so that you'll eat more slowly.

Hold the bread. Ask the waiter not to bring the bread. Or take one roll and send the basket back, says Harvey.

Skip the mixed drinks. Alcohol tends to wake up your appetite—and put your self-control to sleep. So don't drink alcohol before your meal, says Ralph W. Cygan, M.D., clinical professor of medicine and director of the weight-management program at the University of California, Irvine, College of Medicine.

Try a smaller portion. Ask the waiter for a smaller portion, says Harvey. For instance, you can request a meal half the size.

Don't entrée right away. When eating out, have a small bowl of noncreamy soup, such as minestrone, or a small salad before making a decision on your entrée, says Dubner. That way, you won't be as hungry when ordering.

Or don't order it at all. Instead of ordering an entrée, order an appetizer, says Harvey.

Start low, end high. Eat your vegetables first, then eat your starches, like potatoes and bread, and leave the highest-calorie and fattiest items like meat for last, says Dubner. That way, you'll fill up on the lowest-calorie items and feel too full to finish the high-calorie foods.

Don't worry about detours. Every once in a while—for instance, at Thanksgiving—you will stuff yourself. Don't feel guilty. "You are not going to get lost when you take a detour—as long as you don't keep slapping yourself across the face," says Harvey. You will get lost, however, if you continually berate yourself, she says, because then you will feel so bad about yourself that you'll keep eating.

Top 50 Low-Fat Foods

Regardless of how wholesome a food is, if it doesn't please your palate, you won't eat it. But good taste and good nutrition don't have to be mutually exclusive. There are countless ways in which you can satisfy your hunger without one iota of guilt. Now all you have to do is choose.

Here are 50 top low-fat foods, rated by a random sampling of 100 health-conscious women chosen by the writers of this book. Where appropriate, the choices are critiqued by Toni Ferrang, R.D., owner of Food for Thought Nutrition Consulting in Burlingame, California.

1. Angel food cake. "Great!" Ferrang says. "Make it even better by topping it with cut-up fruit and some fat-free or low-fat yogurt."

2. Apples. Our survey takers loved apples for their crunch and portability. They're a good source of fiber, too, Ferrang notes.

3. Bagels. "Just keep in mind that a typical bagel-shop bagel has 200 to 350 calories," Ferrang says. "You'd be better off eating half of one with some fruit."

4. Baked potato chips. They taste better than previous attempts at low-fat chips, and they aren't as greasy as regular chips. Even better, Ferrang adds, some brands have only 1 gram of fat per serving.

A Smoothie That Stops Cravings

This drink is loaded with essential vitamins, minerals, fatty acids, protein, and fiber. It's a great way to cut down on food cravings because you're giving your body the nutrients it needs.

Just put the following ingredients into a blender, mix, and drink: 1 cup of rice milk; 1 cup of soy milk; 1 cup of apple juice, orange juice, or other fruit juice; 1 banana; 4 strawberries; 1 teaspoon of blackstrap molasses; 1 tablespoon of aloe juice; 1 tablespoon of black cherry juice concentrate; 1 tablespoon of powdered "green" formulation (an herbal combination available at most health food stores); 1 to 2 tablespoons of powdered brewer's or nutritional yeast; 1 teaspoon of raw, organic bee pollen (loose, not in tablets or capsules); and 1 tablespoon of flaxseed oil.

Be creative. Experiment with proportions to taste. Freeze the bananas or strawberries for a thicker, colder drink.

5. Baked potatoes. "To get the fiber, eat the skin," Ferrang says.

6. Bananas. "A banana is the easiest thing in the world to stick in your bag and carry to work or wherever," observed one woman who participated in the survey.

7. Beans. These fiber-rich legumes won kudos for their versatility. "And they give you substance without weight," noted another survey participant.

8. Berries. Blueberries, raspberries, and strawberries are all low-calorie and practically fat-free, and they're loaded with vitamins and minerals, Ferrang says. Try them semifrozen—kind of like Popsicle bites.

9. Brownies. The low-fat kind, of course. "If you combine a low-fat brownie with a piece of fruit, you have a good snack," says Ferrang.

10. Cantaloupe. "It's low-fat and loaded with betacarotene," Ferrang notes.

11. Carrots. Many women said they like to keep carrots handy—washed, cut up, and ready to eat. "A great taste that takes the edge off my appetite," said one respondent.

12. Cereals. "I love cereals because they're really crunchy, and I can get the sweetness I like," offered one woman. She thinks Cheerios lead the pack for flavor.

13. Chocolate syrup. Great for chocoholics since it has plenty of flavor but no fat. Ferrang recommends mixing it in skim or 1% milk for a healthy treat.

14. Corn on the cob. "A great choice," comments Ferrang. One woman recommended seasoning it with spices instead of the usual butter and salt.

15. Cottage cheese. Many survey takers offered ingenious ways of enjoying this old diet staple. One respondent suggested adding herbs such as chives for a super-easy dip or spread. Another said she added cottage cheese to tomato soup for an interesting mix of flavors.

16. Couscous. "Serve this grain with lots of veggies for a more nutritionally rounded meal," Ferrang suggests.

17. Crackers. You have to be very careful with crackers, Ferrang says. "You can easily eat the calorie equivalent of three or four slices of toast." Be sure to choose a fat-free or low-fat version, she adds.

18. Cupcakes. The low-fat varieties can cure a craving for sweets quite nicely. "But be aware that you're getting virtually no nutritional value for the calories you're consuming," Ferrang cautions.

19. Fig or fruit bars. Great to satisfy a sweet tooth.

20. Frozen yogurt. No food in the survey evoked as much passion as this one. Women rhapsodized about their favorite brands and flavors, from fat-free peach to low-fat Death by Chocolate. And all agreed that it tastes even better than ice cream. Frozen yogurt isn't the same as "regular" yogurt, however, and doesn't supply the amount of calcium that its namesake does, Ferrang says.

21. Graham crackers. Just as with "regular" crackers, you can overdo it with graham crackers quite easily, Ferrang notes. Still, she says, they're better than cookies.

22. Grapefruit. "I love the tart, fresh flavor of a grapefruit—even though peeling one sometimes takes a while," one respondent wrote. It's worth the time, Ferrang says, since the fruit is rich in vitamin C.

23. Grapes. They taste great frozen.

24. Hot chocolate. Make it with skim milk. It turns out really creamy, and it's a great chocolate fix. Choose a fat-free, sugar-free mix to save calories, Ferrang suggests.

25. Ice cream. Fat-free and low-fat varieties of ice cream hold their own against the real thing, the women agreed. Ferrang says to try topping it with fruit to make it more nutrient dense—and to keep you from going for a second serving.

(continued on page 116)

50 Ways to Shave 100 Calories

If you eat just 100 extra calories a day—that's two chocolate sandwich cookies—you'll be up 10 pounds in a year. But
you can satisfy that cookie craving if you *cut* 100 calories
from someplace else. Here are 50 painless ways to do it.

1. Instead of 1 cup of low-fat granola with raisins,
   have 1 cup of raisin bran.
2. Have a large caffè latte with fat-free instead of
   whole milk.
3. Eat half of a 4-ounce bagel with an orange rather
   than the whole bagel.
4. Put 1 tablespoon of mustard on a sandwich, not 1¼
   tablespoons of mayo.
5. Instead of 2 slices of cheese pizza, have 2 slices of
   veggie pizza (no cheese).
6. Order 2 slices of cheese pizza instead of 2 slices of
   pepperoni pizza.
7. Top your tossed salad with 3 tablespoons of fat-free
   ranch dressing instead of 2 tablespoons of the real
   thing.
8. Try a Boca Burger or Gardenburger instead of a
   regular hamburger.
9. Have a cup of steamed rather than fried rice with
   Chinese vegetables.
10. Put 1 less tablespoon of butter on your baked
    potato.
11. Have ½ cup of macaroni and cheese and 1 cup of
    broccoli.
12. Eat only half of that slice of chocolate fudge cake
    with icing.
13. Instead of 6 cups of theater-style microwave pop-
    corn, have the same amount of low-fat, butter-fla-
    vored microwave popcorn.

14. Spread 1 tablespoon of all-fruit jam on your pancakes rather than 1½ tablespoons of butter.
15. Instead of whole milk and eggs for French toast, use fat-free milk and egg whites.
16. Munch 1 ounce of baked mini pretzels instead of 1 ounce of pecans.
17. Snack on an orange and a banana instead of a candy bar.
18. Steam asparagus rather than sauté it in 1 tablespoon of butter or oil.
19. Replace 3 bacon slices with 3 slices of Canadian bacon.
20. Have 1 cup of home-style baked beans, not 1 cup of beans with franks.
21. Use 3 teaspoons of dijonnaise condiment instead of 4 teaspoons of mayonnaise.
22. Eat ½ cup of steamed fresh broccoli, not ½ cup of broccoli in cheese sauce.
23. Replace 1 cup of caramel-coated popcorn with 2½ cups of air-popped.
24. Stuff celery sticks with 2 tablespoons of fat-free cream cheese instead of 3 tablespoons of regular cream cheese.
25. Have two chocolate chip cookies instead of five.
26. Replace a 12-ounce can of cola with a 12-ounce can of diet cola.
27. Thicken cream sauce with 1% milk and cornstarch instead of butter and flour.
28. Have 3 ounces of steak instead of 4½ ounces.
29. Grill a cheese sandwich using cooking spray instead of margarine.

(continued)

50 Ways to Shave 100 Calories (cont.)

30. Replace 1 cup of chocolate ice cream with ⅔ cup of fat-free frozen yogurt.

31. Snack on 2 ounces of oven-baked potato chips instead of regular.

32. Instead of 1 cup of macaroni salad, eat 3½ cups of spinach salad with 2 tablespoons of low-calorie dressing.

33. Have 1 tablespoon of peanut butter on your sandwich instead of 2.

34. Order a sandwich on cracked wheat bread instead of a croissant.

35. Snack on ½ cup of fruit cocktail in water instead of 1 cup of fruit cocktail in heavy syrup.

36. Dip chips into ½ cup of salsa instead of ¾ cup of jalapeño cheese dip.

37. In tuna salad, use 1 tablespoon of mayonnaise instead of 3 tablespoons.

38. Use 2 tablespoons of light pancake syrup, not 2 tablespoons of regular.

39. Top pasta with 1 cup of marinara sauce instead of ¾ cup of alfredo sauce.

26. Italian ices. Sweet and refreshing—a perfect summertime treat, respondents said. But watch the sugar content, Ferrang advises.

27. Licorice. A number of women applauded the chewy texture of this low-fat sweet. But licorice also packs a hefty amount of sugar, Ferrang warns.

28. Mixed greens. Many supermarkets now carry ready-to-eat mixed greens that have already been washed and cut up. Dress up your greens healthfully with lemon juice, balsamic vinegar, and a dash of soy sauce, Ferrang suggests.

40. Stop tasting as you cook. The following "tastes" have 100 calories: 4 tablespoons of beef stroganoff, 3 tablespoons of homemade chocolate pudding, 2 tablespoons of chocolate chip cookie dough.

41. Eat ¾ cup of pudding made with fat-free milk rather than 1 cup of pudding made with whole milk.

42. Snack on a papaya instead of a bag of chocolate candies.

43. Munch on 1 cup of frozen grapes instead of an ice cream sandwich.

44. Eat two meatballs instead of four.

45. Choose one serving of vegetarian lasagna instead of lasagna with meat.

46. Eat two Kellogg's Nutri-Grain bars instead of two Kellogg's Pop-Tarts.

47. Replace one large flour tortilla with one 6-inch corn tortilla.

48. Eat one hot dog, not two, at a baseball game.

49. Order your Quarter Pounder without cheese.

50. Shred 2 ounces of fat-free Cheddar on nachos instead of regular Cheddar.

29. Oatmeal. A classic comfort food for many women. "Stick with plain oatmeal that you can season yourself," Ferrang advises. "The flavored varieties (in the packets) have a lot of sugar."

30. Oranges. This citrus superstar supplies lots of vitamins and minerals—especially vitamin C—for hardly any calories or fat, says Ferrang.

31. Pasta. Your best bet is to downsize the portion of pasta and add lots of veggies, Ferrang says.

32. Pears. One woman described them as "low-fat art."

33. Peppermint patties. "You get the satisfaction of eating chocolate without overindulgence," said one woman. "And they come in minis, which is the perfect serving size since they're loaded with sugar," Ferrang says.

34. Peppers. Votes for this veggie ran the gamut from fresh bell peppers to spicy pickled peppers. It's the crunch factor that seems to have won the women over. And as Ferrang points out, peppers have lots of vitamin C, too.

35. Pickles. "I like to eat garlic dill pickles when I get home from work," one woman said. "They don't spoil my appetite for dinner, and they have just a few calories."

36. Popcorn. This snack got great accolades. Most women went for the air-popped kind, though some favored low-fat microwavable varieties. Popcorn is higher in fiber than most snacks, Ferrang adds. You can flavor it with spices or with fat-free butter spray.

37. Pretzels. Pretzels defuse cravings by delivering a one-two punch of salt and crunch. Most have no fat, Ferrang adds, and you can get them without salt, which really is better for you.

38. Prunes. They're filling without being fattening, and they give you an energy boost.

39. Pudding. Chocolate pudding made with skim milk, to be exact. Ferrang suggests opting for the sugar-free mix to save on calories.

40. Raisins. Munch on these for healthy doses of fiber, iron, and vitamin C, Ferrang says. Your sweet tooth will get a quick fix, too.

41. Refried beans. The low-fat or fat-free kind, of course. They're just as spicy and filling and satisfying as the lard-laden kind, but with none of the fat.

42. Fat-free milk. A great way to get your calcium. If you shy away from skim, try it with a shot of chocolate syrup.

43. Sorbet. It's a good alternative to full-fat ice cream, but keep an eye on those calories from sugar, Ferrang advises.

44. Strawberries. For a real treat, buy them in season and add them to low-fat cereal with skim milk.

45. Sweet potatoes. Skip the butter or sour cream. If you want, Ferrang says, you can add a little honey or orange juice for flavor.

46. Tomatoes. "In the summer, you can eat them just like an apple," said one woman. And they're packed with vitamin C, Ferrang says. Sprinkle tomato slices with fresh basil and pepper, then add a splash of olive oil or even a little feta cheese.

47. Tortilla chips with homemade salsa. "Wonderful, as long as the chips are baked," Ferrang says. "Add chopped peppers, onions, and mushrooms for extra flavor." The veggies provide bulk, too, so you'll feel full on fewer chips.

48. Watermelon. It's refreshing and thirst quenching—food and drink all in one.

49. Whipped topping. Several survey takers nominated whipped topping as the best medicine for an aching sweet tooth. If you must eat it, stick with the fat-free version, Ferrang advises.

50. Yogurt. You'll go for the creamy texture of fat-free and low-fat yogurt. Add fiber to this healthy treat by slicing some fruit on top, Ferrang suggests. Other favorite toppings include cinnamon, low-fat granola, and Grape-Nuts cereal.

Natural Fat Burner #2: Water

When weight-loss specialist Donald Robertson, M.D., wants to convince a patient who doubts the fat-burning powers of plain old *eau de tap*, he says this: Give it a week, and you will lose weight.

Does this sound like echoes of a once popular jingle for a quick weight-loss shake? Don't worry. Yes, you can get fast results with water. After 1 week of upping their water consumption to 3 quarts a day, Dr. Robertson's patients often lose up to 5 pounds. But unlike commercial quick fixes, water isn't a gimmick but rather an essential element of weight loss.

"Although most of us take it for granted, water is quite possibly the single most important catalyst in losing weight and keeping it off," says Dr. Robertson, medical director of the Southwest Bariatric Nutrition Center in Scottsdale, Arizona.

Our bodies are between one-half and four-fifths water, depending on the amount of lean body mass. That means that if you weigh 150 pounds, you're probably toting around close to 100 pounds of it.

In the course of a day, the average couch potato loses 2 to 3 quarts of water, depending on the climate, says Dr. Robertson. Your goal is to replace that lost fluid by drinking 8 to 10 glasses (8 ounces each) of water per day. Bump up that amount when you're physically active, when it's hot outside, or when you're traveling by plane. For every extra calorie you burn, you'll need an additional milliliter of water, or about 1 cup for every 240 calories you burn. And if you're overweight, your body's metabolic needs are greater, so have one additional glass for every 25 pounds of extra weight.

Here, specifically, is how water can help you lose weight and improve your health.

Fuel for Your Fat Burners

Besides having no calories, what makes water the number one weight-loss drink? For one thing, water naturally suppresses your appetite by filling your stomach up so that you eat less. It also helps your body metabolize stored fat and clear your system of wastes, Dr. Robertson says.

Here's why: Your kidneys depend on water to do their job of filtering waste products from your body. In a water shortage, they need a backup, so they turn to your liver for help. Your liver is responsible for mobilizing stored fat for energy. But if the liver has to do some of the kidneys' work, it can't operate at full throttle.

As a result, the liver metabolizes less fat. That means more fat remains in your body, resulting in less weight loss, says Dr. Robertson.

Even slight dehydration, especially the kind caused by taking diuretics, can cause a 2 to 3 percent decrease in your resting metabolic rate, says Wayne Askew, Ph.D., director of the division of foods and nutrition at the University of Utah in Salt Lake City. Since your resting metabolic rate—the number of calories burned when you're doing nothing—accounts for most of the calories you burn daily, even a small drop in it may have a significant long-term effect.

The bottom line is that when your body gets the water it needs to function optimally:

- Your body burns more fat.
- Fluid retention is alleviated.
- You feel less hungry.

A Liquid Energy Booster

Meeting your daily water quota could make you feel more energetic and more alert than a kid on caffeine, according to Susan Kleiner, R.D., Ph.D., affiliate assistant professor of nutrition at the University of Washington in Seattle and coauthor of *Power Eating*.

Water is the most abundant compound in the human body, filling virtually every space in your cells and the space in between them. Every organ and bodily function depends on it. But when you don't drink enough, your

Think Twice about That Cappuccino

Some specialty coffees are like liquid dessert. A typical 16-ounce cappuccino—*grande*—has 180 calories and 9 grams of fat. In comparison, 16 ounces of regular coffee with 1 tablespoon of fat-free milk has 15 calories and no fat.

For a summertime refresher, try a frosty mug of fat-free milk with a splash of coffee. You'll get about half the calories of a cappuccino and a fraction of the fat. As a bonus, you'll get 302 milligrams of calcium.

cells start drying out. To quench their thirst, they start sucking fluid out of the bloodstream, leaving your blood sludgy, like olive oil left in the refrigerator. As a result, your heart has to pump harder to push the blood through, which can tire you out.

You don't have to lose much fluid to become mildly dehydrated. Losing fluid equal to just 1 to 2 percent loss of body weight can affect your performance. Not getting your daily dose of this neglected but essential nutrient also increases your risk for developing everything from the common cold to certain types of cancer.

To tell if you're getting enough fluid to keep you in tip-top shape, check the color of your urine. It should be the color of straw, Dr. Kleiner says. If it's dark yellow or has an odor, you need to drink more water.

Go for the Goal

So how tough can it be to drink the right amount of water? Well, since so many of us don't do it, it's obviously tougher than it looks. Here's how to make it easy.

Make a water plan. Put together a schedule that reminds you to drink, suggests Dr. Kleiner. By the time you feel thirsty, your body has already lost 2 percent of its fluid, so it's important to drink before you're thirsty.

"You need to have a water plan, just like you have a food plan," she says. Drink a couple of cups when you first get up and throughout the day. Skip it in the evening so you don't have to get up at night.

Be sure to have water with every meal. Keep a pitcher of cold water in the fridge and another on your desk at work so that you're less tempted to drink coffee. "Since the thirst mechanism isn't a good one for maintaining hydration, I like to use visual cues, something kept right in view that's going to remind me," she adds.

Measure it out. Fill a bottle or pitcher with your daily water allotment and keep it on your desk at work or on the kitchen table at home. "Your goal is reached when the pitcher is empty," says Elizabeth Somer, R.D., a registered dietitian and the author of *Age-Proof Your Body*.

Perk it up. Some folks just don't like the taste of water, especially what comes out of the tap. Try adding a twist of lemon or lime, mixing in a little fruit juice, or getting one of those filtration systems that not only improve the taste but also take out contaminants. Or you can buy bottled water. "The point is, find water that you like," says Dr. Kleiner.

Quench your hunger. "Many people don't recognize the difference between thirst and hunger," says Dr. Kleiner. When her patients wake up in the middle of the night hungry, she suggests that they drink a glass of water first and wait 10 minutes to see if they're still hungry. Before the time's up, they're back catching their Zzzs.

Drink two glasses of water before every meal. Besides keeping you hydrated, Dr. Robertson says that drinking two glasses of water can make you feel less hungry, possibly reducing your food intake and aiding weight loss.

Is Your Water Safe to Drink?

Bottled water has become such a cliché in this country that some restaurants put silver holders on their tables for the plastic containers. It's particularly popular with women, who are 23 percent more likely to drink bottled water than men are.

"It's the ultimate health beverage," says Gary Hemphill, vice president of the Beverage Marketing Association in New York City, which tracks the bottled water industry.

What about Fluoride?

Kids aren't the only ones who need fluoride. "It's important for adults, too," says Susan Kleiner, R.D., Ph.D., affiliate assistant professor of nutrition at the University of Washington in Seattle and coauthor of *Power Eating*. "Our teeth actually remodel themselves throughout our lifetime, just like our bones, so you must have fluoride."

If you use a water filter (like a Brita), rest assured: It doesn't filter out the fluoride. And some bottled-water manufacturers add fluoride to their products.

"There are no calories, no additives, and the bottle is portable, so it can be taken just about anywhere."

At least 25 percent of bottled waters sold in this country are nothing more than purified tap water, says Mike Miller, general manager of the bottled water division of NSF International, an independent, not-for-profit company based in Ann Arbor, Michigan, that evaluates bottled water and water filtration systems. The FDA has three separate regulations covering its production, and there has never been a single disease outbreak caused by bottled water in the United States.

The same can't always be said of public water. Although many experts, including Miller, say that the United States has one of the safest public water supplies in the world, problems can, and do, happen. Over the years, isolated incidents have occurred involving contamination by parasites, gasoline additives, *Escherichia coli* bacteria, pesticides, and lead that occasionally turn up in some water systems.

Most water is disinfected with chlorine, the same stuff that keeps your swimming pool crystalline. But some studies

What's in Bottled Iced Tea?

A typical 16-ounce bottle of lemon-flavored iced tea packs a walloping 200 calories, nearly 11 teaspoons of sugar, and 48 milligrams of caffeine. A better choice: A cold glass of sparkling mineral water with lemon contains no calories, no sugar—and no caffeine.

have found a slight association between chlorine by-products in drinking water and some cancers. A study of 28,237 Iowa women found a slight increase in colon cancer among women who drank chlorinated water, but, says Timothy Doyle, an epidemiologist with the Centers for Disease Control and Prevention, the results were very weak.

To learn how safe your local water is, read the Consumer Confidence Report for your local water supplier, available in local libraries and schools. You should also receive a copy of the report each year with your water bill. Or check out the Environmental Protection Agency's Web site: www.epa.gov.

When Bottled Is Best

Choose bottled water over tap water in the following cases.

You prefer the taste. Even if it's just municipal water in that bottle, manufacturers usually use extra filtering, reverse osmosis, and other processes to purify water and rid it of the chlorine taste, Miller says.

You have a compromised immune system. Bacteria that would simply send most of us to the bathroom a few extra times could send you to the hospital.

Other Sources to Consider

In reality, the chances of your drinking nothing but water all day are about as slim as a supermodel. So here's what you need to know about other sources of fluid.

Coffee, tea, and other caffeinated drinks. They are diuretics—that is, they step up urination. If you drink 3 cups of coffee a day, in that same time period you could lose up to 2.4 pounds of water, nearly 2 percent of your body weight.

Strawberry-Watermelon Slush

Think of it as liquid ambrosia. Keep a supply of strawberries and watermelon cubes in the freezer for quick drinks and you'll have no trouble getting your recommended 9 cups of fluid a day. Plus, the fruit has lots of vitamin C, fiber, and other nutrients. Calcium-fortified orange juice gives an extra boost of the bone-strengthening mineral.

    4 ice cubes
    6 frozen strawberries
    2 cups frozen seedless watermelon cubes
    ¾ cup calcium-fortified orange juice
    1 tablespoon lime juice

In a blender, combine the ice cubes, strawberries, watermelon, orange juice, and lime juice. Blend until smooth.

Makes 3 cups
Per 1½ cups: 112 calories, 2 g protein, 26 g carbohydrates, 0 g fat, 0 mg cholesterol, 3 g dietary fiber, 6 mg sodium

The more you habitually drink caffeinated and alcoholic drinks, the less likely you are to realize that you are thirsty. If you must drink tea or coffee, switch to the decaffeinated kind. Keep in mind, though, that they still

Drinks You Should Dodge

Don't be fooled by beverages that bill themselves as healthy or a dieter's friend. Here's how to come out ahead.

Limit diet sodas. Many contain sodium, which makes you retain water, and caffeine, which lowers blood sugar and can leave you feeling hungry. Keep your consumption to two or less a day. Opt for noncaffeinated varieties. And match each soda with a large glass of water to flush the sodium out of your system.

Check the water for calories. Many "sparkling waters" or "flavored waters" have more sugar and calories than regular cola.

Save the sports drink for a marathon. They're not necessary for the everyday exerciser—and they deliver big helpings of calories. If you exercise moderately, water is your best fluid replacement.

Eat the fruit. Fruit juice has vitamins, but it's not the best slimming drink. Half a cup contains 45 to 80 calories. Instead, drink water—and eat the fruit. You'll get fiber, which keeps you full longer.

Be careful of coffee. Plain coffee contains minimal calories (5 to 15), but its regular companions—cream, milk, sugar, syrup, chocolate, and whipped cream—are another story. For instance, a tall caffè mocha can pack as much fat as two slices of coconut custard pie. Limit yourself to 1 to 2 cups of coffee a day, and leave out the fatty extras. Many coffee shops will substitute 2% or fat-free

contain some caffeine. To reach your water quotient for the day, caffeine-free herb teas are a better choice.

Beer, wine, or liquor. Alcohol depresses production of the antidiuretic hormone (ADH), which usually tells the

milk for whole. To add flavor without calories or fat, sprinkle on some cinnamon or use flavored beans.

Watch the mixed drinks. They can deliver from 100 to 250 or more calories. So don't exceed one standard-size drink a day. Start with a nonalcoholic beverage since many people guzzle their first drink the fastest. Once the low-calorie liquid has filled you up, have your alcoholic drink.

Order your drink with the lowest-proof alcohol available, ask for a tall glass and more mixer, and specify half a shot of alcohol. Make sure the bartender uses club soda and not higher-calorie soda like 7Up or Sprite. When ordering milk- or cream-based drinks such as Kahlúa-and-creams, toasted almonds, and White Russians, ask for fat-free milk instead of whole or cream.

Develop dry taste. Dry wines contain less sugar than sweet wines. You'll save about 15 calories a glass with Cabernet, Merlot, and Chardonnay, instead of sweet ones such as Niagara and Ravat.

Don't fear beer. Wine has fewer calories, but it's also less filling, so you may drink more than one glass. If you like beer, go for light or nonalcoholic.

Be late. When going to parties where alcohol and food will be served, show up late to avoid the prime eating and drinking hour. And whatever you do, don't stand next to the food.

kidneys to reabsorb water. Without ADH sending its messages, the kidney snoozes and water loss increases. If you drink a 5-ounce glass of wine, you will pass almost the same amount as urine.

Milk. Fat-free milk is 90 to 99 percent water and has just 86 calories a cup, not to mention that it is a significantly better source of calcium than mineral water.

Juice. It's fine if part of your daily liquid quota comes from juice, provided you watch the sugar.

Stick to juices that are nearly all fruit juice, and dilute them with water to reduce calories and improve your fluid intake. Avoid soda: A regular cola has about 150 calories and the equivalent of 9 teaspoons of sugar—about as much as a candy bar. Plus, the dark-colored sodas—both diet and regular—are high in phosphorus, which some studies have shown can leach calcium from the bones.

Sports drinks. These usually have about half the calories of juice and soda. But be careful: The sodium in sports drinks actually enhances thirst, so you'll want to drink even more. "Unless you are sweating a whole lot—as when you exercise for an hour or more—you don't really need these concentrated beverages," explains Dubner.

To make your own sports drink, combine 8 ounces of water (avoid carbonated water, which can make you uncomfortable during or after exercise), 1 teaspoon of lemon juice, ¼ teaspoon of salt, and 4 teaspoons of sugar. Mix well.

Food. Some foods are basically just rearranged water molecules. Lettuce, watermelon, broccoli, and grapefruit are all more than 90 percent water. Carrots and cottage cheese weigh in close behind with 88 percent and 79 percent, respectively.

Water-based food is good for about 35 percent of your daily water requirement.

Your Daily Water Plan

Along with the suggestions offered earlier, consider these tips when developing your personal water plan.

- Never walk by a water fountain without stopping, says Dubner. Figure that 10 big gulps equals 1 cup of water.
- Squeeze lemon or lime wedges into tap or bottled water to give it extra zing—and yourself an extra dose of vitamin C and antioxidants.
- Make sure that you include water any time you have a snack, says Dubner. Maybe even choose salty snacks like pretzels that will make you thirsty.
- Start meals with soup. They're mostly water.
- Fill up your water glass or bottle every time you get up to go to the bathroom. Remember: water out, water in.
- Flavor water by freezing fruit juice in ice cube trays and adding a couple to a glass of water.
- Drink on schedule. Write it on your calendar or program the alarm on your watch to beep every hour. Each time you are reminded, drink a cup of water.

Natural Fat Burner #3:
Aerobic Exercise

Just for a moment, let's play make-believe. Pretend that two 150-pound women lie on couches for 24 hours. Pretend that one woman is made entirely of fat, the other made entirely of muscle.

The woman made of fat would burn about 300 calories during that long, lazy day. The woman made only of muscle would burn about 5,250 calories.

Granted, no one is made entirely of fat or muscle. There are also bones to consider, as well as various other body parts, such as the brain and liver. And lots of water. So the example above serves only to illustrate a point: Muscle burns many more calories than fat. A pound of muscle burns at least 35 calories a day; a pound of fat burns about 2.

The Fat-Burning Power of Muscle

"The more muscle you have, the more calories you burn," says Robert Girandola, Ed.D., associate professor of exercise science at the University of Southern California in Los Angeles.

Muscle burns so many calories because muscle works so hard. Every time we move, we use muscle. Muscle moves our skeletons, allowing us to walk. Muscle opens and closes our jaws, letting us chew. Muscle makes our throats contract and expand so we can swallow. Muscle even makes our hearts beat and blood vessels constrict and expand. At any given time of the day, we use plenty of muscle. During a game of thumb wrestling, for example, your thumb alone works at least nine muscles.

And even while we sleep, muscle stays busy. Muscle continuously rebuilds itself by replacing and synthesizing protein, says Wayne Westcott, Ph.D., strength training consultant in Quincy, Massachusetts, for the national YMCA.

Fat, on the other hand, burns so few calories because it does so little. Fat sits there. It sits on the backs of our arms, on our rear ends, along our stomachs, even around our ankles. It sits. It rests. And it waits. It waits for some day when some muscle complains, "I'm hungry. Feed me!" And then fat sacrifices itself. It breaks down into fatty acids and travels through blood to the hungry muscle or organ. Fat is food in a human piggy bank.

The Problem with Fat

We do need some fat. The body uses fat to make cell membranes, to keep us warm, to transport vitamins, and to run the nervous system, menstrual cycle, and reproductive system. In fact, at least 15 percent of a woman's body should be fat.

The problem is that many women carry too much fat—30 percent or more. For health and weight maintenance, women should aim to keep their fat levels ideally between 20 and 25 percent, says Katherine T. Thomas, Ph.D., assistant professor of exercise science and physical education at Arizona State University in Tempe. The other 70-plus percent of the body would then be made up of what experts call lean body mass: muscles, bones, organs, and water.

Without exercise, keeping fat levels between 20 and 25 percent becomes a losing battle for most women. A combination of the natural aging process and inactivity causes women, on average, to lose about 5 pounds of muscle every decade. That's 175 fewer calories a day that a woman burns each decade after adulthood. That may not sound like much, but it adds up. By the time we hit our forties, we're burning 350 fewer calories a day than we did when in our twenties. And by our sixties, we use 700 fewer calories.

Less muscle means more fat. The slower metabolism caused by less muscle makes the average woman gain about 10 pounds of fat per decade. Ten pounds of fat takes up more space than 10 pounds of muscle. Compare a pound of shortening (pure fat) with a pound of fillet of beef (pure muscle), for example. The pound of shortening is larger. A body that loses muscle and gains fat gets larger and larger and larger, says Dr. Thomas.

Aerobic Exercise: Weight Loss for the Long Run

If you have ever stopped to add up the numbers of calories burned, you might falsely conclude that aerobic exercise does little for weight loss. A half-hour of moderate aerobic exercise will probably burn what seems like a measly 300 calories. Yet you need to burn 3,500 calories to get rid of a pound of fat.

If you exercise three times a week, you burn 900 calories. So you must exercise for 3½ weeks to burn just 1 pound.

By comparison, eliminating nearly 1,000 calories a day by cutting back on food would seem faster and easier than

Two Fat-Burning Myths to Ignore

Myth #1: You must work out for at least 20 minutes to burn fat.

Myth #2: Strenuous exercise does not burn fat.

Both myths are based on the same half-truth, says Mildred Cody, R.D., Ph.D., associate professor of nutrition and dietetics at Georgia State University in Atlanta. Our bodies burn a combination of carbohydrates and fat for energy. For the first 20 minutes of exercise, our bodies burn mostly carbohydrates. After 20 minutes, they start burning fat. During mild exercise, our bodies prefer to burn fat and conserve carbohydrates. During vigorous exercise, our bodies prefer to burn carbohydrate and conserve fat.

The myth is the belief that burning fat causes more weight loss than burning carbohydrates, says Dr. Cody. To lose weight, you need to burn *calories*. It doesn't matter whether the calories come from carbohydrates or fat. Our bodies must eventually replace whatever calories we burn during exercise. And that replacement usually comes from stored fat, she says.

Vigorous exercise, however, does tend to build muscle faster than moderate exercise. So a program of mild to moderate exercise will result in faster weight loss in the beginning, while a vigorous program will result in more weight loss down the road when the increased muscle speeds up the metabolism.

trying to burn the same amount through exercise. By severely limiting the calories you take in, you can lose 2 pounds or more in 1 week instead of in 7. And, in fact, that's what a lot of women try to do, says William Joel Wilkinson, M.D., medical director of the division of epidemiology and clinical applications at the Cooper Institute for Aerobics Research in Dallas.

But in the long run, crash dieting doesn't work. Losing more than 2 pounds a week will peel off muscle as well as fat. That slows your metabolism, which will eventually result in a weight-loss plateau—you'll stop losing weight, despite your efforts, says Dr. Wilkinson. And you can't starve yourself forever. Once food intake resumes, the body adjusts and the pounds return.

Slow weight loss, on the other hand, conserves your muscle. And, when combined with aerobic exercise, the exercise stimulates your muscles to develop and grow. So your metabolism stays the same.

What's the Best Time to Work Out?

"You can find a good reason to exercise at any time of the day," says Susan W. Butterworth, Ph.D., director of wellness services for the occupational health program at Oregon Health Sciences University in Portland. "The best time to exercise is the time that fits into your schedule the best." That increases your chances of maintaining your exercise habit, she says.

So if you enjoy getting up ½ hour earlier than usual, sliding an aerobics video into your VCR, exercising, and then showering and going to work—then mornings are your best time to exercise. If you find you have a spare ½ hour between the time you get home from work and the time you need to cook dinner—then the late afternoon is your best time. If you feel most energetic during your lunch hour—then noon is your best time, says Dr. Butterworth.

The best time is *your* time.

If you made no other lifestyle changes, your 3-day-a-week aerobic program would permanently take off 15 pounds or more in 1 year. That's still faster than the rate that most women put on weight—1 pound a year.

The Right Exercise at the Right Pace

The aerobic part of your exercise equation should include walking, swimming, cycling, and other options. To make aerobic exercise work for you, experts offer the following caveats.

Less pain means more gain. Many women have the misconception that aerobic exercise has to be hard, says Dr. Wilkinson. After all, we do refer to it as working out. Those misconceptions date to the 1970s, when the popular phrase "no pain, no gain" was thrown around with abandon. At that time, experts thought that exercise had to be more regimented and strenuous to produce results. But today experts say that even mild to moderate physical activity can lead to substantial health benefits. Plus, moderate exercise causes fewer injuries than vigorous exercise and is much more pleasant for many people, he says. The new recommendations are not meant to replace the old guidelines but to complement them. The idea is not to stop running or going to the gym if you are already active; the idea is that activity is good for your health at whatever level—so get out there and get moving.

Move slowly to lose quickly. Exercising at a lower intensity seems to take off inches faster than exercising at a higher intensity, when you burn the same number of calories. When researchers studied women who exercised vigorously for a shorter time versus women who exercised mildly but for a longer time, they found that after 12 weeks on the program, the mild exercisers lost 1.2 inches from the waist, while the vigorous exercises lost only a fraction of an inch. Both groups lost the same amount of fat, says Mildred Cody, R.D., Ph.D., associate professor of nutrition and dietetics at Georgia State University in Atlanta. But the vigorous exercisers gained more muscle. And that may be why they weighed more on the scale and lost fewer inches, she says.

Though more muscle probably means greater weight loss in the long run, Dr. Cody prescribes moderate exercise at first. "I would start someone out at a lower intensity and a longer period of time because I think that helps you to change behaviors," she says. "A lot of people go into this wanting to look better, and they are going to see these inches lost as being a pretty good indicator of what they are doing." Also, you have more chance losing weight with mild exercise because you are more likely to do it. Mild exercise is usually more enjoyable for beginners or people who have been sedentary, she says.

Be picky. Before you begin your aerobic program, put some effort into selecting your aerobic activity. What's best? "Whatever you can stick with is going to work," says Peggy Norwood, an exercise physiologist, president of Avalon Fitness, and former fitness director of the Duke University Diet and Fitness Center, both in Durham, North Carolina.

Choose something that you enjoy, says Dr. Wilkinson. It doesn't matter if you inline skate, ski, run, or play hopscotch. You want to make sure to pick something that you can do for at least 30 minutes, three to five times a week.

Start with 5 minutes. Don't worry about exercising for the entire recommended 30 minutes, especially if you are really out of shape. Start with a time that's comfortable, like 5 minutes. Then gradually increase the amount of time to 30 minutes. That way, you can avoid injuries, aches, pains, and other setbacks, says Norwood.

Don't Believe the Scale

The scale is probably the least accurate measure of your weight-loss progress. "Women who are exercising may not lose that much weight on the scale. But they will find their clothes are looser because they have replaced fat with muscle," says Katherine T. Thomas, Ph.D., assistant professor of exercise science and physical education at Arizona State University in Tempe.

Muscle weighs more than fat. But it's more compact. So exchanging a pound of muscle for a pound of fat will make you look slimmer, says Wayne Westcott, Ph.D., strength training consultant in Quincy, Massachusetts, for the national YMCA.

When it comes to health, experts are focusing less on how much you weigh and more on how fat you are. Fatness is measured by the percentage of fat you have to lean body mass (muscle, bones, organs, and so forth). By such standards, someone who weighs 120 pounds but with 35 percent fat could actually be considered fat. And the same woman at the same height who weighs 140 and has only 15 to 18 percent fat could be considered lean.

"Some women are not overweight. But they look out of shape because they have potbellies. Rather than lose weight, they need to exercise," says Alan Weismantel, a physical therapist for Health South in Hanover, Pennsylvania.

You can determine your fat status by getting your body composition tested (at most health clubs, doctors' offices, and university sports medicine departments). Women should try to keep their percentage of fat below 30 percent, says Dr. Thomas.

Weighted Workouts Work Wonders

Resistance training builds muscle much the same way that life builds wisdom. In life, we start out innocent. Then various things stun us—friends gossip about us, our neighborhood associations hike their fees, our husbands forget our anniversaries. But eventually, we get used to such happenings, and they don't stun us anymore.

Muscle building is much the same. First, we lift a moderate weight seven or eight times—what's called a set—until we can't lift it anymore. The muscle gives up under the pressure.

But overwhelm that muscle enough times and it gets used to the activity by building protein and expanding muscle fibers. The muscle rises to the occasion—and eventually the weight doesn't feel heavy anymore.

In one very large study, women lost 3½ pounds of fat for every 2 pounds of muscle that they built. Though that's only a 1½-pound difference on the scale, the change will show up more dramatically on your body. Muscle is more compact than fat. So even if every pound of fat was replaced with a pound of muscle—that is, you lost no weight on the scale—you would still shrink in body size.

Other than helping us to burn more calories and making us look better, resistance training is an integral part of a fitness program for yet another reason. Just as it stuns muscles into growing, resistance training also stresses bones, making them stronger, and especially strengthens the joints. That will protect you from injury in the aerobic part of the program. "There's nothing like a knee or ankle injury to ruin your weight-loss program," says Robert McMurray, Ph.D., professor of sports science and nutrition at the University of North Carolina at Chapel Hill. "This type of injury really sabotages weight loss: You can't walk, jog, or even be active at work and around the house. So you can actually end up gaining weight."

Think "Action" All Day, Every Day

Dish washing. Playing Twister. Tossing a Frisbee. Bread kneading.

You might not think of cleaning your house, playing games with your children, and baking as exercise, but they all burn more calories than sitting in your recliner. They help create an active lifestyle. And that is crucial for controlling weight.

"We're seeing more overweight people today than at any time in history. Yet we are not eating any more than people did in the 1950s," says Dr. Girandola. "The problem is, we rarely walk anywhere. Most of our leisure activities involve staring at a screen, and we have every conceivable laborsaving device to minimize our activity at home and at work."

Slowly eliminating our dependence on laborsaving devices is one of the easiest ways to live a more active life, says Dr. Girandola.

Here are some things to consider doing without.

- Electric can openers
- Electric car windows
- Elevators
- Escalators
- Power steering
- Riding lawn mowers

This doesn't mean that you have to go back to life in the 1800s and start churning your own butter, says Dr. Girandola. Rather, you need to consciously start making your life more active.

"Women who clean house for a living tend to be relatively healthy because housecleaning is hard work," says Dr. Thomas. "It certainly is not what most people would consider exercise. But activity is critically important."

Try to fit in a total of 30 minutes of activity most days of the week, says Elizabeth Howze, Sc.D., associate director for health promotion in the division of nutrition and physical activity in the National Center for Chronic Disease Prevention and Health Promotion at the Centers for Disease Control and Prevention in Atlanta. For instance, climb stairs for 5 minutes, walk around the supermarket for 15, and vacuum for 10. On the days when you do ½ hour straight of an activity like aerobic dance, continue to look for opportunities to get more activity during that day. Remember, the more you do, the greater the benefit, she says.

Eventually, leading an active life will become second nature. You won't have to make an effort to do it. But at first you'll need to do some planning, says Susan W. Butterworth, Ph.D., director of wellness services for the occupational health program at Oregon Health Sciences University in Portland. She suggests sitting down with a family member, friend, neighbor, or coworker and making a long list of fun things that you can do that don't involve your couch or bed. "The activity can be educational or social. It doesn't have to be a formal exercise session," she says. For instance, your list might include the following:

- Taking your family or a friend to a botanical garden or arboretum
- Going to the zoo
- Tossing around a Frisbee with your children, a friend, or your pet
- Playing fetch with your dog
- Going shopping

The list can involve home life, work life, or social life. Once you have your list completed, plan at least one activity a week, says Dr. Butterworth.

Though the number of calories you burn will depend on how intensely you do your activity and for how long, you can expect to burn 150 calories a day, or about 750 more a week, by adding in ½ hour of aerobic activity on most days, according to Dr. Howze.

Below are some of the most popular and enjoyable fitness activities. Pick your favorites, and use them as the basis for your shape-up program. Experts evaluated the cost and convenience of the following exercises as either low, medium, or high. To do that, they compared the exercises with walking (lowest cost, highest convenience) and downhill skiing (highest cost, lowest convenience).

Aerobics Classes

- **Calories burned:** up to 114 in 15 minutes
- **Convenience:** medium
- **Cost:** medium

For weight loss, an aerobics workout can hardly be beat, says Laurie L. Tis, Ph.D., associate professor in the department of kinesiology and health at Georgia State University in Atlanta. Research shows that aerobic exercise imparts increased feelings of well-being and self-confidence while relieving stress, depression, symptoms of premenstrual syndrome, and sleep problems.

Before you begin, shop for cross-trainer shoes, which provide good cushioning, support, flexibility, and traction for performing the variety of exercises that aerobics workouts entail. If you have high-arched feet, look for a shoe with added shock absorption and more ankle support. If your feet tend to be flatter, look for less cushioning and greater support and heel control.

For a proper fit, allow ½ inch between the end of your longest toe and the end of the shoe. Your shoe should also be as wide as possible across the forefoot without allowing your heel to slip. A well-fitted shoe does not require a breaking-in period. If your feet are blistering after a few days, take the shoes back. Finally, replace your shoes regularly. They lose their cushioning after 3 to 6 months of regular use, making you more susceptible to knee and ankle injuries.

Wear "breathable" fabrics in a blend of cotton and synthetic fibers that whisk sweat away from your body, allowing you to keep cool. If the temperature in your workout area varies, wear clothes in a couple of layers that you can take off or put back on as needed.

Aerobics videotapes are a great way to exercise at home. Look for a workout and music that spark your personal interest. If your time is limited, use 30-minute videos and put a couple of them together at those times when you can do a longer workout. If you're a beginner, decrease the time or the intensity of your routine if it feels too difficult. Don't overestimate what you can do, or you risk getting discouraged right off the bat, says Dr. Tis.

Many aerobics exercises require a degree of motor skill and coordination, which could take time to develop. Start with an introductory class or a videotape workout described as low-impact or no-impact, which means less stress to your joints. As you get comfortable with the exercise program, gradually move into a more advanced workout.

Prepare your body and mind for exercise with a 5- to 10-minute warmup of the muscles you will use during your workout. For example, walk in place to warm up your legs. Follow with "static" (gentle, with no bouncing) stretching of those same muscles.

The talk test is a good, commonsense way to judge whether you're working out at a safe pace, says Richard Cotton, chief exercise physiologist for the American Council on Exercise in San Diego. You should be able to carry on a conversation at the same time you're exercising. If you can't, slow down. Aim for 30 to 60 minutes. If you're an absolute beginner, start out doing only 10 to 15 minutes at a low to moderate intensity level. As you grow stronger, gradually add workout time without increasing intensity.

Most aerobics classes are followed by a few minutes of exercises specific to muscle strengthening. Look for a class that focuses on your "problem areas." Or add toning exercises with light weights to your home workout.

Aerobics Workouts

The best approach to exercise intensity is to work at your own pace, says Lauri Reimer, director of aerobic instructor training for the Aerobics and Fitness Association of America. "In a class, don't worry about keeping up with the people in the front row."

Do 5 leg kicks instead of 10 if that's all you can handle right now. Jump, but skip the arm-reaching part of jumping jacks. Just keep moving. "The point is to do as much as you can and aim for improvement over time," Reimer says.

Monitoring your heart rate can help you ascertain whether you're working out at a safe and effective intensity. For maximum weight loss, work out for 30 to 60 minutes at moderate intensity most days of the week, says Laurie L. Tis, Ph.D., associate professor in the department of kinesiology and health at Georgia State University in Atlanta.

Beginner. 10 to 20 minutes, 3 days a week; target heart rate 60 to 65 percent of maximum

Intermediate. 20 to 30 minutes, 3 to 5 days a week; target heart rate 65 to 75 percent of maximum

Experienced. Minimum 20 to 30 minutes, 3 to 5 days a week; target heart rate 75 to 90 percent of maximum

As few as 3 minutes of moderate movement, like walking, after a workout enables your heart and muscles to slowly return to their normal state, says Dr. Tis.

Bicycling

- **Calories burned:** up to 119 calories in 15 minutes
- **Convenience:** high
- **Cost:** high

Biking is a great aerobic activity if you're overweight because it involves little or no bouncing—your legs spin in a circle, with little impact on your joints.

Biking is also incredibly convenient. You can ride for pure exercise, or you can ride with your husband or chil-

Bicycling Workouts

When you first start to cycle, don't try to conquer hills or ride for a set amount of time, says Edmund Burke, Ph.D., professor of exercise science at the University of Colorado in Colorado Springs and coauthor of *Fitness Cycling*. Instead, choose flat terrain. "You want to feel successful each time you ride, so you look forward to getting on the bike the next time. For the first few weeks, just think of your rides as being a nice, easy way to spend your leisure time."

Your next goal will be to change the intensity of your workout and make it just a little bit longer, perhaps an hour total. "Change one thing in the beginning, such as adding hills or using a higher gear," says Dr. Burke. "And always give yourself some time to recover from the change in intensity before you make another change during the ride."

As you progress, take longer, more challenging rides at least once a week, says Dr. Burke. "You can ride solo," he

dren, commute to work, or bike to the store. If you use a stationary bike, you can read or watch television while you pedal.

But biking does involve fairly expensive equipment. You'll need to buy a bike (outdoor or indoor) or a gym membership.

Biking also has some physical drawbacks. Some outdoor bikes require the rider to hunch over, which can be hard on the back, says Hy Levasseur, an exercise physiologist and director of health education and fitness for the U.S. Department of Transportation in Washington, D.C. That's especially a problem for people who are extremely overweight, he says, and he suggests overweight people buy a recumbent bicycle, which allows them to lean back while riding.

says. "But I think it's helpful to join a biking club and ride with a group. Everyone will be doing the same ride, in terms of intensity and distance, which inspires most people to the next level of fitness."

Beginner. Cycle nonstop for 20 minutes on flat terrain, 2 or 3 times a week for 3 to 4 weeks.

Intermediate. Beginning on flat terrain, cycle fast for 20 to 30 minutes, then include a couple of hills or shift to a harder gear for 5 minutes at a time, without necessarily going fast. Do this 3 times a week until you work your way up to riding comfortably 60 minutes each time.

Experienced. Extend one of your regularly scheduled rides, probably on the weekend, to at least 1½ to 2 times the time or distance of a weekday ride. Vary the speed and intensity as you ride: Climb hills, ride quickly for a few minutes, and use more intensity at other times.

When riding a stationary bike, don't set the resistance so high that you can barely pedal. "A lot of people don't spin their legs around enough, and that's where the aerobic workout comes from," says Nancy C. Karabaic, a certified personal trainer in Wheaton, Maryland. If you're a beginner, aim to ride at 80 revolutions per minute. Once you get in shape, shoot for 90 to 100 revolutions per minute, she says.

When adjusting the seat on a stationary or an outdoor bicycle, make sure that there is a slight bend in your knees. If your legs are too straight, you will hurt your knees. If your knees are too bent, you won't be able to power the bike as well, says Karabaic.

Cross-Country Skiing

- **Calories burned:** up to 150 calories in 15 minutes
- **Convenience:** medium
- **Cost:** high

Simulated cross-country skiing is a great workout for the upper and lower body and easier on your joints than running, but you shouldn't expect it to be the best calorie crusher. You also shouldn't expect to master the machine on the first day since it requires coordinating arm and leg movements.

Unlike outdoor skiing, you needn't concern yourself with boots and bindings. Your feet will be inside toe cups on the machine, so you need only to wear a pair of comfortable cross-trainers or running shoes. Some experts prefer running shoes because their pointier toes fit more snugly in the footholds.

Whether you're buying a machine or using one at the gym, here's what to look for. Ski machines come in two basic types. One, called a dependent system, links the skis with poles that you move back and forth or up and down with your hands. One foot moves forward, and the other automatically moves back. These machines are easy and safe to use, but they aren't as challenging as independent systems and may become boring.

An independent system works each foot separately and uses a cable, rather than poles, that you pull with your hands. This type of machine takes longer to learn, but the independent foot action is smoother and more enjoyable to use. Also, an independent machine forces you to use your upper body, so it gives you a more balanced workout.

Your ski simulator should be sturdy and have separate resistance settings for the legs and arms so that you can increase the tension on either one or both as you become more proficient in the use of the machine. It also should have a mechanism to adjust for arm length. This will enable you to use the machine comfortably regardless of your height. Some machines have electronic monitors that tell you how fast you're moving, how many calories you're burning, how long you've been on the machine, and how far you've traveled.

Although ski simulators can be hard to get the hang of, enthusiasts say they are worth the effort. Establishing a rhythm while moving your arms and legs is difficult. "There's a big learning curve," says Dr. Tis. "It takes practice."

"Start with your legs and get used to that motion—then add the arms. Take it slow. Don't go on the machine and expect to be an expert right away," says Mike Smith, spokesperson for NordicTrack, one of the leading manufacturers of cross-country ski machines. Stick with it, and you'll eventually get the hang of it, he adds.

Cross-Country Skiing Workouts

All cross-country skiers—outdoors and indoors, regardless of skill level—need to warm up before working out, says Steven E. Gaskill, Ph.D., an exercise physiologist at the University of Minnesota in Burnsville, former head coach of the U.S. Nordic Combined and Cross-Country Ski Teams, and author of *Fitness Cross-Country Skiing*. Gently stretch your hamstrings by propping each leg in turn on a low table or stool and bending forward until you feel tightness, not pain, in the back of the leg. Add a few toe touches and shoulder rolls and you're ready to go.

During workouts, beginning skiers should be able to talk easily. If you can't, you're pushing yourself too hard. If you're an advanced skier, you may want to train in intervals, periodically picking up the pace or pushing up hills but always recovering to the point where you can speak in full sentences, with equal amounts of time pushing and recovering, says Dr. Gaskill.

Keep in mind that how hard and how long you work ultimately determines the degree of physical benefit that you get from cross-country skiing. "Long and slow movement,

Elliptical Training

- **Calories burned:** up to 150 in 15 minutes
- **Convenience:** medium
- **Cost:** medium

An elliptical trainer is a near-perfect exercise machine. It looks like a combination treadmill, cross-country ski machine, and stepping machine, and it boasts the benefits of hiking, cross-country skiing, and biking. Working out on the trainer feels like standing on a cross-country ski

for example, can teach your body to burn fat more efficiently, while high-intensity skiing will especially affect your aerobic fitness as well as calorie loss," says Dr. Gaskill. "Most people start out by basically walking on their skis. But even that gives a little more of an upper-body workout than regular walking. Once you learn to glide on the skis and push with the poles, cross-country skiing uses about as much muscle as any activity you could devise."

Beginner. 25 to 45 minutes on a level or gently rolling trail, using the classic skiing technique

Intermediate. 45 to 75 minutes on a prepared trail with rolling hills, using the classic technique or the skating technique

Experienced. 65 to 100 minutes on a packed, hilly trail, using the classic technique or the skating technique; alternate 3 to 5 minutes of high-speed skiing (at the fastest pace you can sustain) with 10 to 15 minutes of recovery skiing (in which your heart rate slows to about 65 percent of maximum)

machine, but instead of your feet moving back and forth, the machine forces them to move around in an oval (or elliptical) pattern.

Using the elliptical trainer doesn't create any impact, so it's easy on your joints. And it's versatile: You can use it to climb or glide. For your effort, you get a calorie-burning workout that pumps your heart like an all-out run without the same stress and strain on the joints in your body. Even though most women burn hundreds of calories on the elliptical machine, they feel as if they're just strolling along.

As a result, you can get rid of unwanted fat without having to push yourself as hard as you do on other machines.

Because your feet don't leave the elliptical trainer's surface, any lightweight athletic shoe will suffice, says Gregory Florez, owner of Fitness First, a personal training company in Chicago and Salt Lake City. Just be sure not to tie the laces too tightly, or your feet will start to feel numb.

To keep your feet dry and blister-free, pair those shoes up with athletic-wear socks of synthetic or cotton/synthetic fiber blends that "breathe," advises Florez.

As with a stationary cycle, resistance on an elliptical trainer determines how much effort it will take for you to keep your feet moving. Ramp levels control how high or low the angle of the ellipse is. For instance, a high ramp mimics hiking, while a low ramp mimics cross-country skiing. Ideally, says Florez, you want to be able to move at a comfortable, moderate speed, interspersed with occasional bursts of high intensity as well as high speeds.

When you first step onto an elliptical trainer, you'll probably start going backward. That's fine for a minute or two, but going backward doesn't work the legs as effectively as forward motion. You will burn slightly more calories by going in reverse, says J. Zack Barksdale, an exercise physiologist at the Cooper Aerobics Center in Dallas, but not enough to make up for the potential strain you're putting on your knees.

Instead, simply place your feet on the footpads and push forward slightly. The trainer will begin to move your legs in the elliptical shape; all you have to do is follow along. The higher the level of resistance, the harder you'll have to push.

While you may be tempted to power your way through the virtual hills and valleys over which the elliptical machine can take you, stay in the midrange of the ellipse at first. Also, people with lower-back problems may find this kind of exercise jarring, so consult your physician before working out on an elliptical trainer.

Getting your balance on an elliptical machine can be a little tricky at first. But bear in mind that you'll burn far more calories if you let go of the handles than if you hang on. Allow your arms to swing freely or try a little of a pumping action.

Elliptical Training Workouts

"At first, start off with 10 minutes of elliptical training at a low intensity," says J. Zack Barksdale, an exercise physiologist at the Cooper Aerobics Center in Dallas. "Do this twice a week for 1 week, then begin to change the workouts. To do this, increase something every week, but don't increase two things at once. For example, in the second week, you could increase the number of times you exercise from two times to three times. Then, in the third week, you might increase your intensity. In the fourth week, you could increase from 10 to 20 minutes. Keep making changes in your workout every week in order to see the most results. And make sure you include other kinds of aerobic activity in your weekly exercise routine, in addition to the elliptical trainer."

Beginner. Two or three times a week for 10 to 20 minutes at a time in a slow rhythm

Intermediate. Two or three times a week for at least 20 minutes, using a preprogrammed workout that doesn't include intervals

Experienced. Two or three times a week, for 20 to 60 minutes of interval training, either preprogrammed or self-directed

It may be easy to get distracted and look around or talk to someone while you're on the trainer, but twisting your torso is a no-no. To keep your knees in line with your feet and avoid injury, always point your head straight ahead.

Jogging

- **Calories burned:** up to 149 calories in 15 minutes
- **Convenience:** high
- **Cost:** low

"If you asked me what was the best single thing that you could do for yourself to help you trim down and lose weight, it would be jogging, provided your hips, knees, and ankles can handle the stress of jogging," says Levasseur.

Jogging uses the muscles of your whole body: your legs to push off and your arms and trunk for balance. Using all

Jogging Workouts

To be sure you're working hard enough (but not too hard), keep track of your heart rate as you jog, says Ellen Glickman-Weiss, Ph.D., associate professor of exercise physiology in the department of exercise, leisure, and sports at Kent State University in Ohio.

To determine your ideal maximum heart rate range— an intensity that's neither too easy nor too hard—subtract your age from 220. Multiply that number by 0.6—that's your lower-limit heart rate for exercise. Next, multiply the same number by 0.9—that's your upper limit.

Make sure your heart rate falls within this range while you exercise. First, take your pulse while walking or marching in place. Place your first two fingers (never your

that muscle translates into burning a lot of calories, about 600 an hour. Which gets to the reason that jogging isn't it ranked *numero uno* in many people's fitness program. In a word: pain. Because jogging puts so much pressure on your joints, you literally run the risk of injury to your ankles, knees, and hips. Almost every expert consulted said that people who are overweight should not run.

Is there any way to avoid injury? Yes, says Alberto Salazar—world-class marathon runner and coach to fellow running champion (and injury-prone) Mary Decker Slaney. Here are the (slow) steps he advises for beginning runners.

1. Start by alternating between 1 minute of walking and 1 minute of running for up to 10 minutes. Do that for 2 weeks.
2. Proceed to 2 minutes of running for every 1 minute of walking, and increase your total time to 15 minutes.

thumb, which has its own pulse) either on the inside of your wrist below your thumb, or below your jaw, next to your windpipe. Count the beats for 15 seconds. To get your heart rate, multiply the count by four. If you find it difficult to take your pulse while exercising, get a sports watch that monitors your heart rate, suggests Dr. Glickman-Weiss.

Beginner. Alternate jogging and walking for 20 minutes a day, 3 to 5 days a week.

Intermediate. Jog 40 minutes at least 4 or 5 days a week.

Experienced. Jog for an hour, up to 5 times a week, not to exceed 30 miles a week. Beyond 30 miles, there is really no extra benefit, and your risk of injury increases.

3. Gradually build up to a nonstop 20-minute jog followed by a 10-minute walk.
4. Then try for a full ½-hour jog.
5. Stay at ½ hour for a few months—even if it feels easy, says Salazar. That will give your joints a chance to get used to jogging.

Rowing

- **Calories burned:** up to 150 calories in 15 minutes
- **Convenience:** medium
- **Cost:** high

Rowing Workouts

Many rowing machines come complete with a digital readout of distance traveled, time elapsed, and calories used so that you can track your progress and intensity level. Heart rate monitors are also available with some models. Machines can also be programmed to time your rest and work times if you want to do interval training.

"When you first start rowing, don't try to go as fast as possible," says J. Zack Barksdale, an exercise physiologist at the Cooper Aerobics Center in Dallas. "You'll tire out too quickly and not burn as much fat as you probably want to. Instead, warm up on a stationary cycle, then come over to the rowing machine and go at a moderate pace for 20 minutes, if you can." Going longer, rather than fast, will burn more fat.

Once you get used to the rower, try to increase your intensity for 30 seconds at a time, then back off for 30 seconds. At first you'll be able to repeat this for only 20 minutes (if that), says Barksdale. But eventually you can try to work your way up to a longer workout of 40 min-

In one study of various exercise machines, scientists found that rowing machines burned about 600 calories an hour at a perceived effort described as somewhat hard. They also work your entire body and don't jar your joints.

The key to using a rowing machine is to put your back into the motion, says Karabaic. She says to start with your knees bent and your arms forward. Then push back with your legs as you keep your arms and back straight. Once your legs are extended, lean back from the hips and pull your arms to your chest. Then sit up, push your arms forward, and bend your knees to the starting position. This instruction is guaranteed to trigger your past-life memories as a galley slave, she says, so be prepared.

utes or so. Be sure to warm up for 5 minutes and stretch your hamstrings and lower back before you row. Cool down for 5 to 10 minutes after rowing. Once your heart rate drops below 90 beats per minute, it is safe for you to stop completely. Barksdale suggests using a treadmill or a stationary cycle for your warmup.

Finally, you'll be ready to keep the pace going longer. Aim for a high-intensity workout of 40 to 60 minutes. Again, make sure that you warm up and cool down.

Beginner. Row for 20 minutes at least twice a week. Keep the resistance light, but not so light that momentum moves you.

Intermediate. Row hard for 30 seconds, then easy for 30 seconds. Try to do 20 to 40 minutes at least 3 times a week.

Experienced. If you are rowing at this advanced level, warm up for 5 to 10 minutes, then keep a steady, high-intensity pace going for 40 to 60 minutes. Do not bend your knees past a 90-degree angle. Cool down. Repeat 4 or 5 days a week.

With rowing, what you *shouldn't* do is as important as what you *should* do.

Don't lock your knees or your elbows when you're at the end of the stroke, says Barksdale. Although your legs and arms will be "straight," you can protect your joints by keeping them loose, relaxed, and slightly flexed.

Use your back and legs equally, rather than focusing on the pulling motion of your upper body. "Your arms and legs should move in a rhythmic, flowing motion as part of the equipment," Barksdale explains.

Finally, don't give up. Learning how to row properly takes a long time, says Holly Metcalf, president and founder of Row as One Institute, a rowing school and camp for women located in South Hadley, Massachusetts. "Rowing appeals to people who like both mental and physical challenge," she notes. "In the beginning, you'll push yourself mentally because you have to learn proper form and technique. The physical challenge of a tough workout will come later on."

Spinning

- **Calories burned:** up to 178 in 15 minutes
- **Convenience:** medium
- **Cost:** medium

Also known as studio cycling, Spinning is basically road cycling brought indoors. It's done on a specially designed workout bike and is set to music or a series of visualizations.

Even if you tried stationary cycling and hated it, you'll love Spinning. For one thing, it simulates riding a bike more than stationary cycling does. A Spinning bike has a weighted wheel, called a flywheel, which picks up speed when you pedal, so you feel as if you're actually going down (or up) hills, or just riding along a country road. You can also stand on a Spin bike in order to climb the "hills" with more power (and thus change the muscles you're working in your legs). Finally, Spinning is a group activity. A certified Spinning instructor leads your ride, making for some of the most intense—and addictive—workouts most women have ever experienced, says Ron Crawford, a certified Spinning instructor from Niles, Ohio, and president of World of Fitness, which operates two fitness facilities.

Spinning bikes include built-in water bottle holders since you're going to need to stay hydrated during the class. Most of the holders will fit a small bottle of water—preferably one with a pop-up spout so you don't have to interrupt your ride to open up your bottle.

Like riding any bike, Spinning can irritate a tender tush (or other sensitive spots). Bike shorts have extra padding in the butt to cushion you. They're available at most sporting goods stores. Some gyms provide bike seats filled with gel, while others expect you to bring your own. Available at sporting goods stores, gel seats have a lot more give than a traditional bike seat.

"Most gyms offer a Begin to Spin class for rookies," says Crawford. "The instructor will show you how to adjust your bike so that you're safe and comfortable as you ride." The bike needs to be adjusted for your height. If the seat is too low or the pedal tension is too high, for example, you may experience knee pain.

Aim for balance between speed (how fast you pedal) and resistance (how hard it is to pedal). You want to keep some resistance on the flywheel; otherwise, it will feel as if your legs are moving out of control.

Although Spinning is a group activity, there is absolutely no competition. "No one can tell at what resistance level you're riding," says Crawford. "And no one will force you to stand when everyone else is standing or to jump if everyone else is jumping." Tune in to the experience of how the ride feels for you, he says, not how you're doing in relation to anyone else in the class.

Spinning Workouts

Even beginner Spinning is intense. You need to take it slow in order to build up your speed, stamina, and endurance carefully, notes Deborah Gallagher, a certified personal trainer and certified Spinning instructor in Vacaville, California. "It takes 3 to 4 weeks before you begin to notice a buildup in the muscles and connective tissues in your legs. While you can do all kinds of rides, it's important to take it slow and not rush through all your different positions."

You can't necessarily anticipate what kind of rides an instructor will offer, says Gallagher. But in general a beginner should stay at low levels of resistance and take the time to get used to the variety of instructors and rides available—seated flat, seated hills, standing hills, running, and jumping.

And remember—no competition!

Beginner. Take Begin to Spin classes twice a week, with no jumping allowed. Keep this schedule consistent for 4 to 6 weeks.

Intermediate. Move on to 3 classes per week. To work your legs, work out at a slightly higher pedaling speed.

Experienced. After 2 to 3 months of steady riding (three times a week), you're ready for the big time: Include jumping and other intense moves like sprinting (high-speed pedaling at light to moderate resistance, as though you're hurrying to finish a race).

Stairclimbing

- **Calories burned:** up to 150 calories in 15 minutes
- **Convenience:** medium
- **Cost:** low to high

Who ever thought that climbing stairs would be the "in" thing to do? Enter the stairclimbing machine—and a whole different way to exercise. It's a great workout for your buttocks, thighs, hips, and calves. And because it doesn't involve bouncing, it's easy on the joints.

Some experts, however, think that stairclimbing may be too much of a good thing because it's so effective in building buttock, hip, and thigh muscles—precisely the places where most women want to lose inches. "It will make your thighs and hips firmer, but they might not get smaller," says Levasseur. To stair-step to slimness, he suggests stair-stepping at low intensities.

Another way to avoid bulky hips is to make stair-stepping only one part of your exercise mix. That way, you will avoid overworking those large leg muscles.

When using a stairclimbing machine, think form, not speed, says Cedric X. Bryant, Ph.D., director of sports medicine for StairMaster L.P. in Kirkland, Washington. Many people set the machine on the fastest motion, thinking they're burning maximum calories. But at that intensity, most people compensate for the super-fast speed by leaning on the console, tightly gripping the handrails, and locking their arms—all of which cut calorie burning by 20 to 25 percent, no matter what the readout on the machine says.

To use the machine correctly, set it at an intensity that allows you to stand up straight and only loosely grip the handrails for balance.

Instead of pushing down on the pedals, try to step up. The pedals are designed to lower at a controlled rate. It's

Stairclimbing Workouts

Although the terms *stepper* and *stairclimber* are used interchangeably, they are two different machines. Steppers work only your lower body. You balance on the handlebars, pushing alternately with one foot at a time. Climbers work the whole body. Whichever machine you're using to get the benefits of stairclimbing, don't try to go all out when you first mount the machine, say experts.

"If you start small and go slow, you'll eventually be able to light up the display monitor on your machine for relatively long, intense workouts," says Cedric X. Bryant, Ph.D., senior vice president of research and development/sports medicine at the StairMaster Corporation in Kirkland, Washington. "The key is to begin with short workouts that are within your capabilities."

Once you're comfortable working out for 20 minutes at a low to moderate intensity, try to begin high-intensity

the stepping-up motion that prevents the pedals from sinking to the floor and provides the workout.

The bigger the step you take, the more calories you will burn. But Dr. Bryant cautions against going for the highest step possible. You want to find the exact stepping motion that is right for you. While it might be comfortable for the person next to you to step up 9 inches, you might be comfortable only with 5, and that's fine.

In fact, Dr. Bryant's final words about stairclimbing machines apply to all the aerobic exercises discussed in this chapter: "The real trick with any type of exercise routine aimed at weight control is that you want to find your comfort zone. That way, you are going to be able to do the exercise longer and more consistently, which will allow you to maintain your body weight or lose weight."

training. To do this, once again you'll have to start slow. Cut down on the number of times per week that you exercise, but increase the level at which you exercise.

Beginner. Five minutes at the lowest level you feel comfortable with—every day, if possible. Work your way up to 20 minutes at this intensity.

Intermediate. Once you can do 20 minutes of exercise every day, cut down on frequency, but increase intensity. Exercise for 2 days on and 1 day off, raising the intensity level every few workouts. Aim for 20 minutes, three or four times per week.

Experienced. Alternate between high and moderate intensity: For every minute of high-intensity exercise, do 2 minutes of moderate-intensity work. Continue for 20 minutes, three or four times a week.

Walking

- **Calories burned:** 100 per mile
- **Convenience:** high
- **Cost:** low

What could be simpler than putting one foot in front of the other? That's all there is to walking. You don't need fancy equipment, a health club membership, or even good weather. Indoors, you can walk on a treadmill or stride around a mall. Outside, the sky's the limit.

Best of all, walking can give you all the rewards of aerobic exercise, but it puts less stress on your knees, hips, and back. A walking routine can help lower your risk of heart disease, reduce your cholesterol and blood pressure, speed up fat loss, and increase muscle tone, says Rosemary Agostini, M.D., clinical associate professor of orthopedics at the University of Washington and staff physician at the Virginia Mason Sports Medicine Center, both in Seattle.

Priority one for all walkers is good shoes. The shoe should bend where your foot bends—at the ball of your foot, not in the middle of the shoe. There should be a thumb's width from the end of your longest toe to the front end of the shoe. If the toe box isn't big enough, your toes will be tingling 20 minutes into your walk. Look for shoes that are lightweight, with a thin heel and a flexible sole. Running and walking shoes with soles that are extremely thick and cushioned are not good for walking. Also stay away from aerobics, tennis, and basketball shoes. Cross-trainers are too stiff and inflexible for walking and don't offer the proper support.

If you need to lose 50 or more pounds or you are relatively inactive, don't overdo it at first. Aim for a daily 20-minute walk at a pace that makes your breathing just a bit labored but doesn't leave you out of breath. "At the end of 20 minutes, you'll probably feel great, as though you could do more—but don't," says Bonnie Stein, a nationally known racewalking instructor and coach from Redington Shores, Florida. "In the first 2 to 3 three weeks of walking, don't go more than 20 minutes per session."

If you can, walk the entire 20 minutes without stopping. But even if you can walk only 10 minutes at a time, you'll get some benefits. Slow down and rest for a few minutes, then begin again.

Plan to walk every day. Even on days when you don't feel like doing it, just get out and walk a few blocks," says

Stein. You'd be surprised at how, once you get going, those few blocks can turn into a mile or more.

If you're an indoor walker, consider buying a treadmill. Stein recommends a motorized version. Set it at a speed that lets you walk comfortably without holding on. When you feel balanced and are used to it, you can increase the speed. Walk on a treadmill for the same amount of time that you would if you were walking outside.

Walking Workouts

Beginners should aim for a level of exertion equivalent to a 6 or 7 on a scale of 1 to 10, advises Bonnie Stein, a nationally known racewalking instructor and coach in Redington Shores, Florida. You should be able to carry on a conversation without being short of breath.

Another way to measure exertion is to monitor your heart rate. To calculate your target heart rate, see "Jogging Workouts," page 154.

Your heart rate should be 102 beats per minute when you walk. As you develop endurance and lose weight, increase your walking time and the intensity by recalculating your target heart rate at a higher percentage or by aiming for an exertion level of 7 or 8.

Beginner. Twenty minutes, 6 or 7 days a week for 2 weeks

Intermediate. Twenty-five minutes, 6 or 7 days a week; increase walking time by 10 percent increments each week until you reach 40 minutes

Experienced. Continue to increase walking time by 10 percent until you reach 45 to 60 minutes, 6 or 7 days a week. If you don't need to lose body fat, you can walk 20 to 30 minutes, 3 days a week, to stay fit.

50 Easy Ways to Burn 150 Calories

Another way to get the exercise you need is to work it into your daily routine. Think of is as putting your body in motion—any kind of motion, says Dr. Howze.

"Consider any activity exercise, whether it is climbing stairs, gardening, or carrying groceries," says Frank Butterfield, a certified fitness trainer in Las Vegas and chairperson of the professional development committee for the American Council on Exercise.

You should stay in motion long enough to burn at least an extra 150 calories on most days, says Adele L. Franks, M.D., assistant director for science with the National Center for Chronic Disease Prevention and Health Promotion at the Centers for Disease Control and Prevention and scientific editor for the 1996 Surgeon General's report on physical activity.

Most moderate physical activities—dancing, walking briskly from room to room, and raking leaves—will burn 150 calories in about ½ hour. So instead of counting calories, you can count minutes, aiming for at least 30 minutes of motion a day, says Dr. Howze.

If you can't get it in all at once, consider amassing your 30 minutes in small chunks of time rather than doing it all in one shot, says Dr. Howze. "Research suggests that women who are trying to lose weight by increasing their activity are more likely to do so when they break up their activities. Think about exercise as something that can be done over the course of the day and that does not require extra time."

For instance, during the next few days, clock yourself every time you climb a flight of stairs, walk, clean, garden, or do any other activity that involves putting your body in motion. Then, at the end of the day, add up your active time. You'll probably find yourself looking for ways to add 5 minutes of activity here and there. Suddenly, exercise will seem easy and enjoyable, says Dr. Howze.

Take Your Pick

Thirty minutes is only a rough estimate of how much motion you need to burn 150 calories (and then only if you weigh 150 pounds). An activity like snow shoveling, for example, burns calories more quickly than an activity like window washing: 15 minutes of snow shoveling equals an hour of window washing.

To ensure that you burn your 150 calories, take your pick from these 50 activities.

- Ironing clothes for 68 minutes
- Shooting pool for 58 minutes
- Canoeing leisurely for 50 minutes
- Cooking for 48 minutes
- Wallpapering for 45 minutes
- Washing and waxing a car for 45 to 60 minutes
- Washing windows or floors for 45 to 60 minutes
- Playing volleyball for 45 minutes
- Ballroom dancing for 43 minutes
- Stocking shelves for 40 minutes
- Playing croquet for 38 minutes
- Cleaning blinds, closets, and shelves for 36 minutes
- Fishing for 36 minutes
- Mopping floors for 36 minutes
- Grocery shopping for 36 minutes
- Walking 1¾ miles at a moderate pace in 35 minutes
- Dusting for 34 minutes
- Vacuuming for 34 minutes
- Playing horseshoes for 33 minutes
- Playing table tennis for 33 minutes
- Gardening for 30 to 45 minutes
- Wheeling yourself in a wheelchair for 30 to 45 minutes
- Shooting baskets for 30 minutes
- Bicycling leisurely 5 miles in 30 minutes
- Dancing fast for 30 minutes

- Doing a country line dance for 30 minutes
- Pushing a stroller 1½ miles in 30 minutes
- Raking leaves for 30 minutes
- Walking briskly 2 miles in 30 minutes
- Mowing the lawn with a power push mower for 29 minutes
- Snowmobiling for 29 minutes

Exercising in Tight Quarters

Will you be stuck on a plane, train, or bus for a while? That doesn't mean you can't exercise. You can work almost every major muscle group in your body without getting out of your seat by doing isometrics, says Robert Lavetta, a fitness trainer in Palm Desert, California, who owns Healthy Lifestyles, a nutrition, fitness, and stress-reduction counseling service. Isometrics involves pushing against static resistance. For a total-body isometric workout that you can do while seated, try this.

1. Put your hands together as if you were going to clap. Your elbows should be out, parallel to the floor. Your fingers should be facing away from your sternum. The heels of your hands and backs of your wrists should rest against your chest. Squeeze your hands together while breathing out. Hold until you finish exhaling and then release. You should feel as though you just worked your chest.

2. Put your hands together as if you were in a praying position. Your fingers should be pointed up and your elbows out, parallel to the floor in a straight line with your wrists. Use your right hand to push against your left hand. Keep your left hand stable. Breathe out as you push. Once you have ex-

- Golfing on foot (no cart) for 26 minutes
- Inline skating leisurely for 26 minutes
- Stacking firewood for 25 minutes
- Snorkeling for 24 minutes
- Bowling for 23 minutes
- Playing leisurely badminton for 22 minutes
- Playing Frisbee for 22 minutes

haled, stop pushing, take a breath, and then do the same movement by pushing against your right hand. You should feel as if you worked your shoulders and chest.

3. Put your palms against the top of your outer thighs. Apply firm pressure and exhale as you slide your hands toward your knees. As you return your hands to their original position, relax and inhale. Concentrate on flexing the back of your arms to work the triceps as much as possible.

4. Put both hands underneath your right knee. As you exhale, use your hands to pull your right thigh and knee toward your chest. Your right leg should act as deadweight. Make sure to use your arm muscles and not your leg. You should feel as though you just worked your biceps.

5. Sit with your knees together and place your hands on either side of them. Exhale and push your legs against your hands to work the outer thigh and shoulder muscles. You can easily reverse this exercise to work the inner thighs. Just put your hands between your knees to provide some resistance and squeeze your legs together as you exhale.

- Scrubbing floors for 20 minutes
- Sawing wood by hand for 18 minutes
- Grooming a horse for 17 minutes
- Backpacking with an 11-pound load for 17 minutes
- Riding a motorcycle for 16 minutes
- Forking hay for 16 minutes
- Twirling a baton for 16 minutes
- Bicycling fast 4 miles in 15 minutes
- Shoveling snow for 15 minutes
- Climbing stairs for 15 minutes
- Doing the twist for 13 minutes
- Snowshoeing in soft snow for 13 minutes

The Fidgeting Factor

The average woman burns 1 to 2 calories a minute while sitting. Veronica Canfield, 31, of San Antonio, however, is not your average woman. As she sits in front of her home computer, she burns more calories by shaking her legs, squirming in her seat, tapping her feet, and twirling a pencil between her fingers. In other words, she fidgets. By doing so, Veronica burns somewhere between 110 and 620 more calories a day than if she sat still, according to one study that measured that calorie-burning potential of fidgeting.

Fidgeting is just one small way to work activity into your inactivity. Here are more than two dozen others, from weight-loss specialists and fitness trainers.

Become an inefficiency expert. When it comes to going somewhere or getting something done, try to be as inefficient as possible. Instead of using a big sponge to wipe up a mess, use a smaller one. Instead of using a mop, get down on your hands and knees and scrub that floor. When cleaning windows, get rid of the laborsaving squeegee and use a rag instead.

Tote more groceries. Instead of trying to lug every grocery bag into the house in one trip, make multiple trips by carrying one bag at a time, says Kathy Mangan, a certified lifestyle and weight-management consultant and a certified personal trainer at the Women's Club, an all-women's health and fitness facility in Missoula, Montana.

Clean to be lean. When cleaning the house, use large, exaggerated movements. Chances are, you'll burn more calories, says Vicki Pierson, a certified fitness trainer and weight-management consultant in Chattanooga, Tennessee. For instance, when cleaning windows, use big arm circles. And when vacuuming, use long, slow rhythmic movements. Switch arms to work both sides of your body equally.

Boycott the car wash. Get out the soap and hose and do it yourself, says Mangan.

Kid around. Rather than popping in a video, play actively with your children or grandchildren. Play catch, jump rope, climb on the monkey bars, push them on a swing, or run foot races. Most anything a child enjoys will give you a good aerobic workout.

Say good morning to your body. Before getting out of bed in the morning, kick down the covers and raise your arms as if you were reaching for the sun. Take a breath and drop your arms forward on the bed toward your legs. Repeat three or four times to get your heart beating slightly faster. Then get out of bed, says Robert Lavetta, a fitness trainer in Palm Desert, California, who owns a nutrition, fitness, and stress-reduction counseling service called Healthy Lifestyles.

Walk a long distance. When answering the phone, scurry to the one that is farthest from you, says Pierson.

Don't use the closest parking lot. To work more walking into your day, park ½ mile away from work, suggests Dr. Cody. "It's a small behavior change that has tremendous positive results."

Rediscover the stairs. Whenever possible, take the stairs instead of the elevator or escalator. If you work on the 108th floor and couldn't possibly walk up that many steps, take the first few flights and then ride the elevator. You can add a few more flights to your workout each day. When walking stairs, walk them as quickly as you can. Or, for variety, take two steps at a time.

Leave the cart in the store. When at the supermarket, carry your groceries to the car instead of using a cart, says Pierson.

Take exercise breaks. During breaks at work, walk the stairs or walk around the building instead of reading the paper or visiting the water cooler, says Pierson.

Earn your inactivity. For instance, if you enjoy reading, don't allow yourself to read your book until after you've walked.

Take a "long cut." Whenever walking somewhere, take the long route, whether you are on your way to the mailroom or to the corner store, says Pierson.

Hike to the ladies' room. Start using a bathroom on a different floor from the one on which you work, or at least one that is farther from your office, says Mangan.

Make dancing dates. Go out with your partner once or twice a month to a dance club or to take dance lessons.

Curl your drink. Whenever you grab a gallon plastic jug from your refrigerator, make it your habit to do a biceps curl with it a few times before opening it, says Lavetta.

Go in circles. While at work, get up every so often and walk two circles around your desk, says Mia Finnegan, a Fitness America Pageant National Champion and Miss Olympia Fitness, who with her husband operates a training service called Tru Fitness in Pasadena, California.

Give up sunbathing. When at the beach, stay active by swimming, wave surfing, renting a rowboat or paddleboat, or playing paddleball, says Pierson.

Get back to basics. If you have a riding mower, switch to a push mower, says Pierson.

Be a Ms. Fix-It. Whenever possible, take on home improvement projects—such as painting and wallpapering—yourself. You will not only get a workout but also save money, says Pierson.

Have a motorized locker room. Designate an area in your car as the "locker room." Keep a pair of sneakers, clean socks, a clean towel, a Frisbee, some tennis rackets, a basketball, or any other items that you think you might use. Then the next time you are out and about with a little extra time, stop at a park and shoot some hoops, take a jog, hit a tennis ball against a wall, or do some other activity, says Pierson.

Be your own squeeze. When driving, standing in line at the deli counter, or waiting at the doctor's office, tighten your butt cheeks, thighs, and abdominals to give your muscles a workout, says Finnegan.

Give yourself a raise. While washing dishes, do toe raises to work your calves, says Tereasa Flunker, an exercise physiologist at ReQuest Physical Therapy in Gainesville, Florida.

Squat, don't bend. When getting clothing out of the dryer, instead of bending over, do a squat to work your leg and butt muscles. Do the same when picking things up from the floor, says Flunker.

Lose control. When you don't have a remote control, you have to get up and walk to the television to change the channel. You also may watch less television, in general, says Norwood.

Get down. When in the house, put on some of your favorite tunes and dance. Dance while walking from the table to the sink. Dance while picking things up off the floor, says Levasseur.

Natural Fat Burner #4: Strength Training

Joyce Stoner's 44-year-old body was beginning to reveal its age. Joyce meticulously watched what she ate, yet unwanted pounds slowly attached themselves to her hips. She regularly sweated to step aerobics, yet found flab on her thighs and a pouch on her tummy.

Joyce knew that she couldn't stop the aging clock, but she wanted to at least slow it down. So she hired a personal trainer to take her through a weight lifting and aerobics routine 2 days a week.

Six months later, Joyce looked in the mirror and liked what she saw. It was as if she had traded in her old body for a new model.

"People had always told me that I had great legs, but I didn't see it," says Joyce, an administrative assistant from New Carrolton, Maryland. "Now I'm noticing that I have great legs. My buttocks are firm. And I just love my arms. Before, I wouldn't wear a tank top. Now I wear sleeveless clothes without hesitation. And my breasts—they seemed small before. After strength training, they look bigger.

"My husband has never said that I needed to lose weight," adds Joyce. "But he's noticed the changes."

Why Strength Training Works

As you age, your metabolism slows. So, like Joyce, you start putting on pounds even though you're not eating more food. In some cases, women might even eat less food—and still gain weight. That slower metabolism is caused in part by an age-related loss of muscle. Well, strength training (or weight lifting, as it is also called) reverses that process. It builds muscle and speeds metabolism, says Wayne Westcott, Ph.D., strength training consultant in Quincy, Massachusetts, for the national YMCA. The result is that you burn more calories—even when you're sleeping. And you lose weight or don't gain any extra.

That's why strength training is such a crucial ingredient of a weight-loss exercise program—it helps speed up the metabolism. Sure, there are other ways to burn calories: lifestyle changes like walking up the stairs instead of taking the elevator or doing aerobic exercise. But only strength training builds the kind of muscle that's needed to give your sluggish metabolism a swift, firming kick in its sagging posterior.

What makes strength training such a powerful muscle builder? And why doesn't aerobic exercise do the same?

In aerobic exercise, the muscle is building predominantly endurance, not strength. When you walk or bike, you are increasing the capacity of your body to deliver more blood to the muscle so that it can work longer without being fatigued, says Morris B. Mellion, M.D., clinical associate professor at the University of Nebraska Medical Center and team physician for men's and women's sports at the University of Nebraska, both in Omaha. But in strength training, the cells of your muscles actually grow. When you ask a muscle to handle more weight than normal and then rest the muscle to let it recover, the muscle cells thicken. The muscle is bigger, firmer.

Building muscle also sculpts the body. A pound of muscle is smaller, firmer, and shapelier than a pound of fat. So as you replace fat with muscle, your body will take on a firmer shape. Try this: Press your finger against the top of your forearm. Your forearm is primarily muscle, so it probably feels pretty hard. Now press your finger against your abdomen, which tends to collect fat. Chances are, your abdomen gives considerably. While fat jiggles, muscle stays in place. And while fat hangs limply, muscle hugs the body, giving you a distinct shape.

Besides making you look better, strength training also makes you stronger. As you progress from fat to firm, you'll find groceries easier to carry, stairs easier to climb, and boxes easier to lift.

Body Sculpting for Women

If you asked a guy why he lifts weights, he would probably tell you that he wants to get bigger. He would say that he wants a chest like a bull, shoulders like a tank, and biceps like bowling balls.

Know any women who want to look like that?

"Women's strength training goals are very different from men's goals," says Mia Finnegan, a Fitness America Pageant National Champion and Miss Olympia Fitness, who with her husband operates a training service called Tru Fitness in Pasadena, California. "The man wants a big, thick chest; a woman wants a shapely breast line. A man wants huge biceps and triceps; a woman wants toned arms. Women want to shrink their lower bodies—shrink their hips, butts, and thighs. Most men don't even care about their legs. They just care about their upper bodies."

Weight lifting can make a guy larger. And the image of the super-muscled male weight lifter can make women shy away from the weight room. Not to worry, though. Only in the rarest of cases do women have the natural ability to build huge amounts of muscle, says Dr. Westcott.

Take Finnegan, for example. At 5 feet 4 inches, she weighs 125 pounds and is around 15 percent body fat. Her arms are sculpted and toned. Her buttocks never jiggle. Her abdomen is enviably firm. But she's feminine and petite. If you saw her walking down the street, you would never suspect that she's a fitness champion who's featured regularly in muscle magazines.

How Dumbbells Got Their Name

Dumbbells aren't shaped like bells. And they're no dumber than a chinup bar. So why do we call this handheld weight a dumbbell?

For the answer, we need to go back in time to the year 1711, when the word *dumbbell* was coined. At that time, bell ringing was a job. A hard, demanding job. A job only a strong person could do.

Problem was, if you needed to ring the church bells just once a week, you didn't ring them often enough to get in shape for the job. And to get in shape, bell ringers couldn't run up to the church tower and ring the bells whenever they wanted to—townspeople would be confused. So during the week, bell ringers began to exercise, using a handheld weight that looked much like the apparatus used to swing a church bell, but without a bell. Because no sound came from the bell-like apparatus, the ringers referred to it as a dumbbell.

When women tell Finnegan they worry that weight lifting will make them big, she asks, "Do you think I'm big?" "No," the women tell her. They say they want to look just like her. So Finnegan puts them on an exercise program that includes weight lifting.

"Nobody ever says, 'I want to get big. I want to look like one of those women in the bodybuilding magazines.' Women want to be tight, toned, and small," explains Finnegan. "Women think that those overly muscular women in the magazines get that way naturally. But those women often have breast implants and drug-enhanced physiques. Few natural woman can gain muscle like that."

So, you won't have biceps like Arnold—or Arnoldette. But you will have firmer muscles and a faster metabolism. Before you begin, however, you need some guidelines for lifting correctly.

Give yourself enough room. Women who begin to lift weights don't give themselves enough elbow room, says Nancy C. Karabaic, a certified personal trainer in Wheaton, Maryland. They tend to keep their arms at their sides and their legs close together to appear ladylike. To train properly, you need to spread out and take up as much room as you need to be comfortable, she says.

Pay particular attention when doing squats and up-right-rowing motions, says Karabaic. To do a squat correctly, you have to stick your butt out, which at first makes many women self-conscious, she says. And upright rowing involves bringing your elbows out to the sides, as if you were trying to jab someone next to you. To do rowing motions correctly, you need to get used to bending your elbows out to the sides.

Start right, start light. Ultimately, your goal for each strength training exercise will be to lift a weight light enough that you can lift it at least 8 times and heavy enough that you can't possibly lift it more than 15 times, says Tereasa Flunker, an exercise physiologist at ReQuest Physical Therapy in Gainesville, Florida, who won the Miss Gainesville title in 1988. But for the first couple of weeks of your weight lifting program, use weights that are slightly lighter than the description above so that you can make sure you use proper form. If you start out with weights that are too heavy, you'll tend to cheat. That is, you'll throw your back into the motion, do repetitions too quickly, or rely on momentum. So in the beginning, concern yourself more with lifting the weights correctly than with lifting heavy weights.

Add weight. Once you're able to comfortably do between 8 and 15 repetitions of an exercise, then you should move up in weight for that exercise, says Karabaic. Some women will feel comfortable doing 8 at the heavier weight, and some will need to wait until they do 15 before adding more weight. In the beginning of your program, you should expect to move up in weight every month to 2 months. After 6 months to a year, however, your muscles won't grow as quickly, so you'll advance in weight more slowly, every 3 to 6 months.

Visualize the exercise. To lift weights correctly, you need to feel your muscles move. Yet some women who are overweight or for any reason uncomfortable with their bodies tend to be out of touch with what it takes to move their bodies, says Kathy Mangan, a certified lifestyle and weight-management consultant and a certified personal trainer at the Women's Club, an all-women's health and fitness facility in Missoula, Montana. So, at first weight lifting may feel foreign.

Visualization can help overcome that awkwardness and help you lift correctly, says Mangan. Before you actually start the strength training exercises on the pages that follow, picture yourself doing the motions. In particular, think about what parts of your body you will use to do the motion correctly and how that might feel.

Don't lock your joints. When doing any exercise, make sure that you don't straighten your elbows or knees so much that you lock your joints. If you do, you'll end up putting weight on the joint instead of on the muscle, possibly causing elbow or knee pain, says Karabaic.

Straighten your wrists. Though you don't want to lock your elbows or knees, you do want to keep your wrists straight, says Karabaic. Otherwise, you may end up with wrist or forearm pain.

Breathe. Don't forget to breathe when lifting weights. Breathe out while lifting the weight and in while lowering it, says Karabaic. Don't hold your breath.

Choose Your Weapon

You can use quite a variety of strength training exercises to both sculpt and strengthen muscle. You can do a complete routine in about 20 minutes, and it should be done three times a week.

Weight machines. Most often found at fitness centers, weight machines employ weights and pulleys or other forms of resistance to work specific muscle groups in specific ways. They offer a controlled workout, taking you through a safe range of motion with constant resistance throughout the entire motion.

Since you don't have to worry about dropping a heavy weight on your head or neck, weight machines are somewhat safer than free weights—dumbbells and barbells. But many machines are designed for the average male body. So unless you're 5-foot-7 or taller, you may find yourself constantly trying to adjust the machine and still never quite feeling comfortable. Don't blame your technique or know-how. Most likely the machine does not fit you properly.

So, for short women, machines may not be the best option, says Karabaic.

Resistance bands. Sold in many sporting goods stores and medical supply stores, stretchy, oversize rubber bands are an inexpensive way to begin a strength training program. To work your arms, legs, and various other muscle groups, you simply stretch the oversize rubber bands in various directions. Commercial brand-name resistance bands are sold in sets, with different amounts of tension in each band. So as one resistance band becomes too easy, you can progress to a more-difficult-to-stretch band.

Resistance bands are convenient: They're easy to store, and you can even take them with you on vacation. But the bands can be unwieldy. As you pull on the band in a circular motion, such as when doing a biceps curl, you'll feel more tension at some points than others, making the movement feel jerky. Also, you need to do more repetitions with resistance bands than you would with dumbbells or a barbell to get the same workout, says Karabaic.

Dumbbells and barbells. Free weights might be your best bet. Dumbbells and barbells are nothing more than hand-held rods with varying amounts of weight at each end, offering many of the same benefits as weight machines. Dumbbells come in pairs, one for each hand. A barbell is longer—you lift it with both hands.

You can get a good workout using dumbbells alone. They're fairly inexpensive and convenient for home use (between workouts, you can store them under a bed).

Getting Set

For a good strength training workout, you'll need various sizes of dumbbells and some sort of a bench. Experts offer these tips for getting equipped.

Buy varying sets of weights. Because different muscles will be stronger than others, you'll need more than one pair of dumbbells. Buy sets of 3-, 5-, and 10-pound dumbbells. Later, as you become stronger, you'll probably need heavier dumbbells. But most beginners don't need anything heavier than 10 pounds, Flunker says. If, however, you find that 10 pounds is too light, don't hesitate to get heavier weights, she says.

Shop secondhand. You can save money on dumbbells by going to a secondhand sporting goods store, such as Play It Again Sports; by scouting garage sales; or by offering to buy lighter weights from bodybuilders who have moved on to heavier levels, says Flunker.

Go for comfort. Unlike treadmills, stairclimbers, and other exercise machines, buying free weights doesn't require a lot of research or comparison shopping. Dumbbells haven't evolved much since the day of their invention, says Mike May, spokesman for the National Sporting Goods Manufacturers Association in North Palm Beach, Florida.

Your main objective is to find dumbbells that are comfortable to hold, says Mangan. Dumbbells vary in length and width. You'll probably feel more comfortable with shorter dumbbells. The longer the dumbbell, the more unwieldy, she says.

You also want a comfortable bench. Some are wider than others. When at the store, lie on the bench to make sure it is wide enough to support your body, says Mangan. You don't want your shoulders or sides to hang over the edge to the point that you feel as though you'll fall off. Also, some benches are taller than others. Make sure that your feet can comfortably touch the floor when you're lying down, she says.

Make do with water jugs. If you aren't ready to purchase dumbbells, you can use plastic gallon milk jugs filled with water, says Molly Foley, an exercise physiologist and director of ReQuest Physical Therapy. A 1-gallon milk jug filled completely with water weighs about 8½ pounds. How much water you use depends on how much weight you intend to lift. Experiment to determine how much water is right for you. You'll probably have to add water or dump some out as you go from one exercise to the next, she says.

Improvise a bench. For beginners, a piano bench, padded picnic table bench, or other rectangular object can suffice as a strength training bench, says Foley. Make sure that your bench allows you to lower your elbows below body level so you can do bench presses and similar exercises, she says. Lying on the bed or the floor won't work.

Slip on the gloves. You can get through your routine without them, but you'll feel more comfortable with a pair of weight lifting gloves. Gloves help you grip the weight securely and prevent calluses.

Staying Limber

Many weight lifting exercises tend to shorten the muscles, which makes you less flexible, says Flunker. Regularly stretching will elongate those muscles, reduce any soreness, lower your injury risk, and give you a greater range of motion. Try to do the following stretches before and after each weight lifting session, in the order given, and do each one three times, holding each stretch about 10 to 20 seconds, she says.

Shoulder circles. Start with your shoulders relaxed, then slowly rotate them backward until you feel loose. Then change directions, rotating them forward.

Shoulder blade squeeze. Stand with your hands clasped behind your back. Lower your shoulder blades by pulling your clasped hands down and lifting your breastbone.

Then raise your clasped hands toward the ceiling as high as you can. Your body may bend forward. Hold for about 20 seconds and then relax.

Chest stretch. Stand in a doorway with one foot a few inches in front of the other for balance. Extend your arms to the side, placing your hands, palms flat, against each wall along the doorway. Lean forward so that you can feel the stretch. Hold for about 20 seconds. Then vary the stretch by moving your hands higher and lower on the walls.

Back flex. Lie on your back. Using your arms, pull one knee to your chest. Hold for 20 seconds, then release. Repeat on the other side.

High Weights, Low Reps? Or the Reverse?

One piece of misinformation might confuse your early weight lifting efforts. Women who work out might tell you that doing a lot of repetitions at a low weight will prevent you from getting big.

They are partially correct. High repetitions at a low weight will build up muscle endurance instead of muscle strength, which means your muscles won't grow as much. Problem is, you are defeating the purpose of your entire weight lifting program if you choose the high-repetition workout. You want your muscles to grow in strength and size to boost the number of calories you burn a day. You are better off doing fewer repetitions with more weight, building more muscle, and burning more calories to burn off more fat, says Wayne Westcott, Ph.D., strength training consultant in Quincy, Massachusetts, for the national YMCA.

Back stretch. Get down on the floor on your hands and knees like a baby beginning to crawl. Your lower legs and thighs should form a 90-degree angle at your knees. Your back should be straight and your arms extended straight down directly under your shoulders. Lower your buttocks toward your heels. (Don't let your hands move out of position.) You will look like a cat stretching. Feel the stretch through your spine. Hold for 20 seconds.

Hip flexor stretch. Get down on one knee, like someone making a marriage proposal. Keep both knees at 90-degree angles. Then perform a pelvic tilt: Keeping your chest upright, lean forward until you feel a stretch in the leg that has the knee on the floor. Hold for 20 seconds and then repeat on the other side.

Hamstring stretch. Lie on your back with your left knee bent and your foot on the floor, the right leg extended straight up at a 90-degree angle to the floor. Flex your right foot. Use your hands to pull the extended leg toward your chest. Hold for 20 seconds. Repeat with the right leg bent and the left leg lifted.

Thigh stretch. While standing, put your left hand on a wall for balance. With your right hand, reach behind you and grab the ankle of your right leg so your foot comes as close as possible to touching your buttocks. Do not lean forward or allow your back to arch. Hold for 20 seconds. Repeat on the other side.

Calf stretch. With one leg in front of the other, about walking distance apart, push against a wall as if you were trying to push it down. Keep the calf you are stretching straight and its knee straight while the other knee is bent and lunging forward in front of you. Keep your heels on the floor and body straight so that you feel the stretch through the calf of your rear leg. Hold for 20 seconds. Repeat on the other side.

Forward neck stretch. Sit or stand with good posture. Bring your chin as close as you can to your chest. Hold for 20 seconds.

Side neck stretch. Sit or stand with good posture. While keeping your face forward, tip one ear toward the shoulder on the same side. Hold for 20 seconds. Repeat on the other side.

Side stretch. Hold your arms straight overhead and clasp both hands together. Lean to one side without leaning forward or backward. Hold for 20 seconds. Repeat on the other side.

A Firm-Body Workout

For allover body toning, follow the workout below, suggested by Michael Pollock, Ph.D., exercise physiologist and professor of medicine and exercise science at the University of Florida, with help from Gainesville exercise physiologists Tereasa Flunker and Molly Foley. The routines that comprise this workout target the chest, shoulders, neck, back, arms, legs, and buttocks, in that order.

When doing the program, follow these guidelines.

Go in order. Do the exercises in the order that they are listed. The exercises are arranged so that you can work the larger muscles in your chest and back before you work the smaller muscles in your arms. The smaller arm muscles assist the large chest and back muscles during exercises such as the bench press and upright row. If you worked the smaller muscles first, you would be too tired to complete the chest and back exercises, says Flunker.

Try to fail. Muscles get stronger more quickly if you work them to failure. That means you have worked your muscle to the point where you can't do a single additional repetition without resting. You want to lift a heavy enough weight so that after 8 to 15 repetitions you have no option but to give up, says Dr. Pollock. Muscle failure makes stronger muscles. As you progress and are comfortable doing between 8 and 15 repetitions, you can do another set or add more weight if using barbells, he adds.

Take breaks. After each exercise, rest for up to 2 minutes before moving on to the next exercise. Rest breaks give your muscles a chance to recuperate and prepare for further effort. When you first begin to work out, you may need to rest for the full 2 minutes before you feel able to do the next exercise. As time progresses, however, you will probably be able to shorten your rest time, says Foley.

Use good posture. Good posture will help you protect your joints and spine from strain, says Flunker. Before each movement, check your posture. Stand with your feet about shoulder-width apart, your knees slightly bent. Let your arms relax at your sides. Lift your breastbone by pulling your shoulders back and down. Roll your pelvis so that your lower back is straight instead of curved inward. Then assume that pose whether you're vertical (standing) or horizontal (lying on a bench), she says. When bending over, keep your back and chest straight by bending from the hips.

Take every other day off. Ideally, you should try to do the routine 3 days a week with at least one day of rest in between workouts. The rest will give your muscles a chance to recuperate, explains Dr. Pollock.

Give the gym a try. Though the following workout involves dumbbells, you can do similar moves on machines at a gym. For each exercise, you'll find the name of the machine you can use at the gym that works the same muscles as that exercise.

Dumbbell Bench Press
Muscles toned: The chest (pectoralis major) muscle around the breast builds up. The flabby back of the upper

arms (triceps) gets hard. The shoulders (anterior deltoids) take on more shape.

What to do: A. Lie flat on a bench with your knees bent and feet flat on the bench. (If you have trouble keeping your balance, you can put both feet flat on the floor.) Hold a dumbbell in each hand, palms forward, with your arms held at a 90-degree angle from your chest—that is, arms straight up.

B. Lower the dumbbells to your chest. Try not to let them wobble as you lower them as far as you can. Then return to the starting position and repeat.

In the gym: Use the chest press machine.

Dumbbell Flies

Muscles toned: The chest (pectoralis major) builds up, helping to accentuate the breasts. The shoulders (anterior deltoids) take on more shape.

What to do: A. Lie on your back on a bench with your knees bent and feet on the bench. Hold the dumbbells above your chest, with your palms facing each other and elbows slightly bent.

B. Lower the weights as you move them out to the side of your body in a wide arc as far as you can. Keep your palms facing each other and elbows slightly bent to reduce stress on the shoulders. Once you have reached the maximum stretch, arc the weights back to the starting position, as if you were giving someone a huge bear hug. Then repeat.

In the gym: Use the arm-cross/butterfly machine.

Dumbbell Press

Muscles toned: The shoulders (deltoids) take on shape, the neck (trapezius) builds up slightly, and the backs of the upper arms (triceps) gets firm.

What to do: A. Sit on a bench with your back straight. Hold the dumbbells in both hands. Bend your elbows to hold the dumbbells even at shoulder level, to the sides of the shoulders. Your palms should face forward.

B. Press the dumbbells overhead. Make sure to keep the weights above your shoulders, elbows slightly bent. Then return to the starting position and repeat.

In the gym: Use the overhead press machine.

Upright Row

Muscles toned: The shoulders (deltoids) and the neck (trapezius) build up slightly and take on shape.

What to do: A. From a standing position, hold dumbbells in both hands with your knuckles facing forward. The dumbbells should be in front of your body below waist level. Your arms should hang down, with your elbows straight.

B. Bend and raise your elbows to pull the dumbbells toward the ceiling. Try to keep the weights as close to your body as possible. Once you have the weights to armpit level, return to the starting position and then repeat.

In the gym: Use the lateral raise machine.

Bent Row

Muscles toned: The back muscles (latissimus dorsi, rhomboids) create a triangle from your shoulders to your waist, tapering your torso.

What to do: A. Kneel on one end of a padded weight bench with your left knee, keeping your right leg slightly bent. Support yourself with your left arm and hold a dumbbell with your right hand. Keep your back slightly arched.

B. Lift the dumbbell until your right elbow is a few inches higher than your back. Remember to keep your back slightly arched and your support leg straight. Return the dumbbell to the starting position and then repeat. After you complete your repetitions, repeat on the opposite side.

In the gym: Use the seated rowing machine.

Back Extension

Muscles toned: The lower back (erector spinae) and buttocks (gluteals) firm up, further toning your torso, waistline, and hips.

What to do: A. Roll up two towels so each is about 2 inches thick. Lie facedown, one towel under your abdomen and the other under your forehead. Extend both your arms on the floor, above your head.

B. Tighten your buttocks as you raise one extended arm and the opposite leg. Your arm should be straight, with your fingers pointing. Your toes should be pointed. Hold for 5 to 10 seconds and then repeat on the other side.

In the gym: Use the Roman chair or hyperextension machine.

Standing Dumbbell Curl

Muscles toned: The upper fronts of the arms (biceps) take on shape and are less apt to jiggle when you move.

What to do: A. Stand with your knees slightly bent and your feet shoulder-width apart. With your back straight and head up, hold dumbbells in both hands, with your arms resting at your sides and your palms facing your outer thighs.

B. Rotate one arm so the palm is facing forward.

C. Curl that arm, bringing the forearm toward your biceps, with your palm facing up. Lower the weight, twist the arm back to the starting position, and repeat on other side. Continue switching sides until you have completed your repetitions. If you prefer, you can also do both sides simultaneously.

In the gym: Use the biceps curl machine.

Seated Curl

Muscles toned: The upper fronts of the arms (biceps) take on shape, improving how you look in sleeveless tops.

What to do: A. Sit on the edge of a bench. Put your feet on the floor, about 2 feet apart. Hold a dumbbell in one hand with your palm facing up. Bend slightly forward and place the hand not holding the dumbbell on the knee on the same side. Then rest the elbow of the hand holding the dumbbell on the thigh, slightly above the knee on that side with the arm hanging down.

B. Curl the dumbbell toward your shoulder, making a semicircle while keeping your elbow on the thigh. Then lower the weight. After you complete your repetitions, repeat on the opposite side.

In the gym: Use the biceps curl machine.

French Press
Muscles toned: Firms up flab on the upper back of the arms (triceps) so that your arms don't jiggle.

What to do: A. With both hands, hold a dumbbell just behind the top of your head. Cup your palms and thumbs around the handle of one end of the dumbbell, elbows extended. Stand straight with your feet shoulder-width apart or sit on the edge of a bench.

B. While keeping your upper arms close to your head, lower the weight behind your head in a semicircular motion until your forearms almost touch your biceps. Return to the starting position, then repeat.

In the gym: Use the triceps extension machine.

Dumbbell Kickback
Muscles toned: Firms the flab on the upper back of the arms (triceps), eliminating jiggliness.

What to do: A. Stand with your knees slightly bent, with one foot in front of the other at a comfortable distance. Place one hand on the bench or on your front knee for balance. Keep your upper torso parallel to the bench. Take a dumbbell in the other hand. Bend that arm and raise your elbow close to your side to shoulder height. Make sure your arm is at a 90-degree angle with your palm facing your side.

B. Your elbow should remain in place as you complete the movement. Press the weight back until your forearm is parallel to the floor. Do not raise it above your body. Hold for a count of two and then slowly return to the starting position. After you complete your repetitions, repeat on the opposite side.

In the gym: Use the triceps extension machine.

Dumbbell Squat

Muscles toned: Tightens, firms, and adds shape to the fronts of the thighs (quadriceps) and the buttocks (gluteals), giving your legs a sleeker, firmer appearance.

What to do: A. Stand with a dumbbell in each hand. Raise the dumbbells to the outside of your shoulders, your palms facing forward.

B. Keeping your head and back in a straight line, bend forward slightly as you bend your knees and lower yourself as if you were going to sit into a chair. Keep your head and neck in a straight line. Lower yourself into a squat as far as you comfortably can, but only until your thighs are almost parallel to the floor. Then raise yourself to the starting position and repeat.

In the gym: Use the leg press machine.

Dumbbell Lunge

Muscles toned: Firms, tightens, and adds shape to the buttocks (gluteus medius, gluteus maximus) and the fronts of the thighs (quadriceps).

What to do: A. Hold a dumbbell in each hand, your arms at your sides and your palms facing in.

B. While keeping your head up and back straight, take a large step forward until your thigh is almost parallel to the floor. Bend your front knee while bringing the trailing knee almost to the floor. Push yourself back to the starting position and then repeat with the other leg.

In the gym: Use a leg press machine that works one leg at a time.

Standing Calf Raise

Muscles toned: Firms, tightens, and adds shape to the calves (gastrocnemius, soleus).

What to do: A. Stand with your toes and the balls of your feet on a step, your heels extended off the step.

B. Keeping your knees slightly bent, lower your heels as far as you can toward the floor or toward the step below.

C. Then rise up on your toes as far as possible. Repeat.

In the gym: Use the standing or seated calf raise machine.

Natural Fat Burner #5: Herbs

Let's face it. If there really were a magic bullet for weight loss, we'd all have taken up target practice by now—and we'd be mighty good shots, too. Even herbalists say that the strongest natural remedies for unwanted pounds are still diet and exercise.

But wait: Don't discount herbs just yet. Chosen and used with care, they can give a sensible weight-loss program an extra edge, according to herbalists. "And under certain circumstances, herbs may make all the difference between success and failure," says Dana Myatt, N.D., a naturopathic physician in Phoenix.

Herbs can promote weight loss in a variety of ways, says Dr. Myatt. Some seem to trick your belly and brain into believing that you just aren't hungry. Others are thermogenic—that is, they rev up the body's metabolism so that it burns calories more quickly. Still other herbs, classified as stimulants, contain substances such as caffeine that speed up certain body functions, such as circulation, heart rate, digestion, and respiration. Stimulant herbs are often also thermogenic. According to herbalists, some of these herbs, like dandelion leaf, green tea, and nettle (described in more detail later) are as safe as, or safer than, prescription and over-the-counter weight-loss drugs. Herbal laxatives and preparations containing the herb ephedra (also known as ma huang), however, have been shown to have serious side effects, says Ara DerMarderosian, Ph.D., professor of pharmacognosy and medicinal chemistry at the Philadelphia College of Pharmacy and Science. Before you take herbs or start any weight-loss program, check with your health care practitioner.

As helpful as herbs can be, however, it's smart to remember the big picture.

First, woman does not lose weight by herbs alone. "Many people believe that there's one magic herb formula that will make the pounds just fall off their bodies," says Dr. Myatt. "No product can do that." So swallowing herbs as you indulge in a diet high in cheeseburgers and pastries or other high-fat, high-calorie foods isn't going to work.

Second, not all herbs have a lasting effect. Diuretics like buchu or uva-ursi, for example, simply rid your body of excess fluid. Water weight returns as quickly as it's lost—overnight.

An Herbal Arsenal

What this all boils down to is that when it comes to using herbs for weight loss, there are no easy answers—and no miracles, either. Still, when teamed with a sensible program of diet and exercise, herbs may work for you, say herbalists. Here's the strategy that's most likely to aid your weight-loss efforts, starting with what you eat and drink.

Crunch, crunch, crunch. Most weight-loss experts agree: If you want to lose weight, eat more foods high in fiber, such as fruits, vegetables, beans, potatoes, and whole grains. High-fiber foods take up more space in your stomach than fat-laden fare, and they tend to be low in fat and calories.

Fiber also stabilizes levels of glucose, or blood sugar, your body's main source of fuel, says Dr. Myatt. Some people produce higher-than-normal amounts of insulin, the hormone that controls the rate at which blood sugar is absorbed by cells. In response to this abnormally high insulin level, the body manufactures more fat cells than normal. The more fat cells you have, the slower your metabolism is likely to become, and the more likely you are to gain weight. Fiber-rich foods don't appear to stimulate the production of insulin as much as do foods made with white flour, such as white bread and baked goods.

Consume 25 to 30 grams of fiber a day, recommends Dr. Myatt. A sample high-fiber menu might include a bowl of all-bran cereal for breakfast (some brands contain as much as 20 grams of fiber per cup), a large fruit salad accompanied by a couple of slices of whole-grain toast for lunch, and a can of water-packed tuna over a mountain of crisp greens and veggies for dinner.

Consider a fiber supplement. Despite their best intentions, "many folks just can't eat 25 grams of fiber a day," says Dr. Myatt. If this sounds like you, consider taking two dietary fiber supplements three times a day, she suggests. Several studies have shown that taking 5 grams of supplemental fiber a day can help women shed pounds. Dietary fiber supplements are available in drugstores and health food stores. And don't skimp on water: Too much fiber plus not enough liquid can equal severe constipation. So swallow the capsules with a full 8-ounce glass of water at the beginning of every meal, she says.

Or take 1 to 2 tablespoons of ground psyllium husks before meals (up to 6 tablespoons a day). Although it's typically used as a laxative, psyllium can also curb a too-hearty appetite, says Silena Heron, N.D., adjunct professor at Southwest College of Naturopathic Medicine and Health Sciences in Tempe, Arizona, and vice president of the Botanical Medicine Academy. Taken before meals with lots of water (two to three 8-ounce glasses), the fiber-rich plant swells like a sponge in your digestive tract. That full feeling in your stomach sends a signal to your brain, telling you not to eat as much. The water is critical to this regimen, cautions Dr. Heron, because if you're dehydrated, psyllium can cause digestive tract blockages.

What's more, several studies on weight loss have shown that diets high in fiber (in these studies it was about 35 grams a day) can reduce by 30 to 180 calories the number of calories absorbed by the body each day. That can add up to 19 pounds a year. One study of 52 people found that those who dieted and also took 7 grams of fiber supplements a day lost nearly double the weight—12.1 pounds versus 6.6 pounds—of those who only dieted.

Pepper your food with cayenne. Add a dash of cayenne pepper (also known as red pepper) or hot-pepper sauce (like Tabasco) to your food several times a day, suggests Dr. Myatt. The active ingredient in cayenne pepper, capsaicin, is a stimulant of saliva, salivary amylase (an enzyme involved in the digestion of starch), and hydrochloric acid, substances that improve the digestive process, she says. "People with sluggish digestion tend to gain weight. Those with efficient digestion tend to maintain a normal weight."

Capsaicin may also accelerate metabolism. In research conducted at Oxford Polytechnic Institute in England, dieters who added 1 teaspoon of red-pepper sauce and 1 teaspoon of mustard to every meal raised their metabolic rates by as much as 25 percent.

Go green. Drink a cup of green tea with a meal two or three times a day, suggests Dr. Myatt. Green tea contains caffeine, a stimulant that revs up metabolism, as well as theobromine, a compound similar to caffeine. Depending on how long it's steeped, a cup of green tea contains 40 to 100 milligrams of caffeine—up to the amount in a cup of coffee. If you're cutting back on caffeine for other reasons, don't drink more than two or three cups.

Green tea has something that coffee doesn't, however: It's rich in vitamin C and flavonoids, compounds that are po-

Weight-Loss Aids to Avoid

"Natural" doesn't always mean "safe." Some natural weight-loss products contain herbs that are potentially dangerous or extremely toxic. Also, because the Food and Drug Administration (FDA) classifies weight-loss products as dietary supplements, not drugs, manufacturers don't need FDA approval to market them. This means that many of these products haven't been proven effective—or safe.

Herbal laxatives. Commonly sold as "dieter's teas," laxative herbs include cascara, senna, buckthorn, aloe, and rhubarb root. These products can cause stomach cramps and diarrhea. If they're overused, your bowels may no longer function without them. Most serious is the fact that these products deplete the blood of the mineral potassium; that can lead to paralysis and irregular heartbeat. At least four women with a history of eating disorders died after misusing these products.

Ephedra. Research on the effects of ephedra, also known as ma huang, on weight loss has been modestly favorable. But at high doses it can raise blood pressure, increase heart rate, and overstimulate the central nervous system, which controls the brain. Since 1996, the FDA has received more than 800 reports of side effects linked with the use of ephedra, including heart palpitations, seizures,

tent antioxidants. These protective nutrients help reduce the risk of illnesses such as heart disease and cancer, especially of the colon. And it promotes weight loss due to its thermogenic effect, which raises metabolism, Dr. Myatt says.

Green tea is sold in health food stores and some supermarkets. It is sold as loose, dried tea leaves and in tea bags, which are easier for some people to use, she says. It also comes in capsule form. The recommended dosage is usu-

stroke, chest pain, and heart attack. This herb has also caused at least two deaths.

Herbal fen-phen. Ephedra is the active ingredient in this "natural" version of the dangerous diet drug combination, fenfluramine and phentermine, which was pulled from the market when it was discovered that it caused heart valve problems. In clinical trials, herbal fen-phen has not been shown to work. Also, its misuse is associated with severe side effects, including nervousness and heartbeat irregularities, as well as death from heart attack and stroke.

Garcinia cambogia. Products containing hydroxycitric acid (HCA), which is obtained from the fruit of the *Garcinia cambogia* plant, won't harm you, but research shows that they may not help you either. HCA is supposed to help control appetite and reduce absorption of fat by the body. A study with 135 overweight men and women, however, showed that HCA had no significant effect on weight loss or fat loss. Given the controversy regarding the effectiveness of HCA, it is probably better to wait until we know more about it, says Connie Catellani, M.D., medical director of the Miro Center for Integrative Medicine in Evanston, Illinois.

ally two capsules three times a day, says Dr. Myatt, but she prefers the tea because "you get a lot more of the antioxidants in a cup than you will in a pill."

Try a five-herb tincture. Schisandra berry (which means "five-flavor seed" in Chinese) grows in the most remote parts of the world. Gum guggul is extracted from a plant related to myrrh, and bladderwrack is a type of brown seaweed. Team these exotic ingredients with some basic herbs, and the result is a remedy that "very gently helps weight loss along by improving metabolism," says David Winston, a professional member of the American Herbalists Guild (AHG) and founder of Herbalist and Alchemist, an herbal medicine company in Washington, New Jersey. Blend the following tinctures (also called extracts) in an 8-ounce or larger bottle (all are available at health food stores): 1 ounce of nettle, 1 ounce of dandelion leaf, 1 ounce of bladderwrack, 2 ounces of guggul, and 2 ounces of Chinese schisandra berry. Take ½ to 1 teaspoon three times a day. (Hold your nose, though: This concoction isn't the most pleasant tasting around, says Winston.)

Bladderwrack is a folk remedy for treating weight problems. Schizandrin, the active ingredient in schisandra berry, gently stimulates metabolism. Dandelion is used by herbalists to boost the liver's secretion of bile, which helps break down the fats in food. Nettle is rich in minerals, which help maintain overall health during weight loss, Winston says. And guggul helps normalize thyroid function, which is sometimes disturbed in overweight people.

See about seaweed. In rare cases, a sluggish thyroid gland can cause weight gain. Seaweed is rich in iodine, a natural thyroid stimulant, says Ellen Hopman, a professional member of the AHG who practices in Amherst, Massachusetts. "It's also a good source of essential trace minerals, such as chromium," she says. Hopman recommends taking seaweed supplements (usually kelp, because of its especially high iodine content) with cayenne supplements. Take one capsule of each once in the morning and once at night, always right after meals. "Never take cayenne on an empty stomach. It won't hurt you, but it will cause a burning sensation," says Hopman.

You'll find kelp and cayenne supplements in most drugstores and health food stores. If you suspect that your

A Beverage to Help Burn Calories

In traditional Chinese medicine, extra weight is an indication that one's digestion is weak. This means that the digestive fires aren't burning hot, so it's easier for the body to transform food into extra water and fat than to convert it into muscle, blood, and energy, says fourth-generation herbalist Christopher Hobbs, a professional member of the American Herbalists Guild, a botanist and licensed acupuncturist in Santa Cruz, California, and author of many books on herbs, including *Handmade Medicines: Simple Recipes for Herbal Health*. To stoke your digestive fires and help shed those pounds, take 1 teaspoon of this bitter tonic, made from a combination of tinctures, in a glass of water before meals.

Chinese Bitter Tonic
- 4½ teaspoons artichoke leaf
- 3 teaspoons ginger rhizome
- 1½ teaspoons angelica root
- 1½ teaspoons cardamom pod
- ¾ teaspoon gentian root
- ¾ teaspoon licorice root

In a small bowl, combine the artichoke, ginger, angelica, cardamom, gentian, and licorice. Store in an amber glass dropper bottle or a dark glass jar.

weight problems are due to a sluggish thyroid or if you're taking thyroid medication of any kind, you should check with your doctor before considering this remedy.

Bladderwrack seaweed also may help you lose weight if your thyroid is iodine deficient, says Dr. Heron. Grind and sprinkle 1 teaspoon over food or add it to soups and stews. A little iodine-rich bladderwrack can rev up a lazy metabolism by stimulating the production of thyroid hormones, she explains. You may find the fishy taste unpleasant, but if you cook the seaweed with grains, soups, or stews, you'll hardly notice it.

Take Asian ginseng. Go for a daily dose of 200 milligrams. Ginseng is known as a feel-good herb to boost vitality, and its ability to regulate blood sugar suggests that it may be useful in helping people lose weight, says Robert Rountree, M.D., a holistic physician at the Helios Health Center in Boulder, Colorado.

"Experts feel that continual high levels of the hormone insulin lead to obesity," he explains. When you eat a starchy meal or drink a sugary beverage (that is, carbohydrates), your blood sugar rises, and your pancreas reacts by releasing insulin to bring it back down. Insulin receptors in the body allow glucose to enter cells, lowering blood sugar levels, explains Dr. Rountree. As we age, these receptors move less glucose into the cells, and the resultant high levels prompt the pancreas to produce more insulin. Insulin then instructs the fat cells to convert the excess glucose and fatty acids into fats called triglycerides, which are stored until needed. As long as glucose levels—and thus insulin levels—are elevated, the fats remain in storage. Too much of this fat results in obesity.

"If you can control insulin levels, maybe you can stem the fat-storing process from the beginning," says Dr. Rountree. He estimates that half of his overweight patients have abnormally high levels of insulin in their blood.

Research shows that Asian ginseng—also known as panax, or Korean or Chinese ginseng—can help correct blood sugar levels. In a study in Finland, 36 people with type 2 (non-insulin-dependent) diabetes who took a daily dose of 200 milligrams of ginseng for 8 weeks lowered their fasting blood sugar levels and lost weight. Even more important, they reported that they felt better and were able to exercise more.

Counter the urge to indulge. When something sweet beckons, squirt a few drops of *Gymnema sylvestre* tincture on your tongue. Used for centuries in Ayurvedic medicine to treat diabetes, this herb, also known as gurmar, can help fend off a craving for sweets. "It has the unusual property of blocking sugary tastes," says Nancy Welliver, N.D., director of the Institute of Medical Herbalism in Calistoga, California. Squirting the tincture directly onto your tongue will block the taste of sugar for about 15 minutes. Look for it in health food stores, says Dr. Welliver.

Sweeten coffee and baked goods naturally. Use a smidgen of stevia, a South American herb. Artificial sweeteners like saccharin and aspartame offer calorie-free alternatives to sugar, but both have been linked with health problems, says Connie Catellani, M.D., medical director of the Miro Center for Integrative Medicine in Evanston, Illinois.

Stevia is a noncaloric herbal sweetener sold as a dietary supplement in health food stores. Since it's 200 to 300 times sweeter than sugar, you need only a pinch to satisfy your sweet tooth, says Arthur O. Tucker III, Ph.D., research professor at Delaware State University in Dover. And, unlike with aspartame, you can also cook and bake with it. Some recipes call for substituting 2 tablespoons of stevia powder for 1 cup of sugar. The extract form is much sweeter, so if you use that, you'll need only about ¼ teaspoon for every cup of sugar, says Dr. Tucker.

Natural Fat Burner #6: Vitamins and Minerals

Shakes, puddings, powders, and grapefruit: Name the diet, and you've tried it, each time hoping it would be the one that works. Then you watched that dread needle on that dreadful scale drift right back up to where you started.

Despite sage advice against dieting from physicians and national experts, we're still doing it. National surveys indicate that 84 percent of women and 77 percent of men "go on diets" when they want to lose weight. And regardless of all of that calorie counting, our national waistline continues to expand, with 33.4 percent of Americans now overweight.

Could it finally be time to throw in the towel and pick up the fork? "No," says Judy Dodd, R.D., past president of the American Dietetic Association. "We just have to be sensible about our diets. Even people who are genetically predisposed to putting on weight do not have to be overweight. There are steps you can take to beat it, such as exercise and nutrition."

Multivitamins May Lend a Hand

So what about vitamins and minerals? What role do they play in a sensible no-diet weight-loss plan? Although the topic is controversial, some doctors believe that multivitamin/mineral supplements, combined with a healthy food and exercise plan, can help. They find that the struggles of overweight people are often brought on by a combination of poor general nutrition and dieting that leaves them feeling fatigued and craving food.

"It becomes like a dog chasing its tail," says Michael Steelman, M.D., vice president of the American Society of Bariatric Physicians. "When people don't feel good mentally and physically, they will often eat sweets to try to make themselves feel better, only to find themselves feeling worse. The first line of defense is getting proper exercise and nutrition."

Unfortunately, given the wide appeal of fad diets, that's easier said than done, says Dodd. "Some of the old fad diets, such as the high-protein diet, are popular again, and people tend to skimp on important dietary elements such as fruits, vegetables, and dairy."

According to diet research, the most popular diets—those emphasizing high or low levels of protein, carbohydrates, and fat—all lead to deficiencies in important vitamins and minerals, particularly vitamins A and C, thiamin, iron, and calcium. And low-calorie diets, even those that are well-balanced, typically lack folate, vitamin B_6, magnesium, and zinc.

"Nutrition is a problem when people restrict calories," says Dodd. "I encourage people to get their vitamins and minerals from natural food sources, but if they go below 1,200 calories, they should consider a multivitamin/mineral supplement with 100 percent of the Daily Values."

In fact, multivitamin/mineral supplements are good for anyone who is overweight, dieting or not, says Donald Robertson, M.D., medical director of Southwest Bariatric Nutrition Center in Scottsdale, Arizona. "Too many overweight people are nutritionally deficient. Supplementation helps keep them healthier."

Aside from multivitamin/mineral supplements, here are some of the nutrients that many experts believe can help you stay healthier and feel better and may even promote weight loss.

Nutrients to Build Immunity

As if the well-documented health risks associated with being overweight, such as heart disease and diabetes, weren't bad enough, some researchers now believe that overweight people have lowered immunity, perhaps because of deficiencies of vitamins and minerals, especially the antioxidants.

Antioxidants, such as vitamins C and E, are important because they protect our bodies against free radicals, unstable oxygen molecules that damage your body's cells by stealing electrons from healthy molecules. Antioxidants offer their own electrons, neutralizing free radicals and protecting cells.

According to a study done in Poland, overweight people may not be reaping antioxidant benefits. Researchers at the National Institute of Food and Nutrition in Warsaw studied 102 overweight women and found that compared with women of normal weight, the overweight women had significantly lower levels of the antioxidant vitamins C and E, as well as of vitamin A, and a higher prevalence of overall vitamin deficiency.

These deficiencies are at least partially responsible for depressing immunity in overweight individuals, leaving them more susceptible to cancer and infectious illness, say some researchers.

And because of abnormal hormone activity, overweight people may also have a greater need for antioxidants than people who are not overweight. Studies show that the excess fat in people who are very overweight drives estrogen production up and testosterone down, a deadly combination that scientists believe could be a major factor in certain female reproductive cancers.

"Overweight people probably need antioxidants more than anybody," says Dr. Robertson. He recommends daily supplements of 1,000 milligrams of vitamin C and 400 international units of vitamin E, along with 25,000 international units of vitamin A. These doses greatly exceed the Daily Values of these nutrients, and vitamin A in particular can be toxic in high doses. Research has found that taking 10,000 international units of vitamin A daily in early pregnancy can cause birth defects. For this reason, that much vitamin A should be taken only under medical supervision, especially if you are a woman of childbearing age. And pregnant women should not use this therapy.

To get more antioxidants through your diet, reach for fruits and vegetables. Those with bright orange coloring, such as sweet potatoes, carrots, and cantaloupe, are rich in beta-carotene (a precursor of vitamin A); broccoli, brussels sprouts, and citrus fruits will give you a burst of vitamin C; and wheat germ and kale are good sources of vitamin E.

Chromium Can Help

It might not be the waist-whittling miracle mineral that some advertisements tout it as, but according to the latest research, chromium picolinate (a supplemental form of chromium) may indeed help build lean tissue and reduce fat in adults who exercise.

In one study of 59 college-age students at Louisiana State University in Baton Rouge, researchers found that women taking 200 micrograms of chromium picolinate a day gained almost twice as much lean body mass as those who did not take the supplements. This effect could result in long-term reductions in body fat since lean body mass burns more calories than fat.

"What makes the effectiveness of chromium more and more believable is that the results we see in humans are so well-documented in animal studies," says Richard An-

Prescriptions for Healing

Some nutrition experts find that overweight people have special vitamin and mineral needs, especially if they're trying to lose weight. Here's what these experts recommend (in addition to a multivitamin/mineral supplement containing the Daily Values of all essential vitamins and minerals).

Nutrient	Daily Amount
Calcium	1,000 milligrams; 1,500 milligrams for postmenopausal women
Chromium	50–200 micrograms (chromium picolinate)
Copper	1.5–3 milligrams (1 milligram for every 10 milligrams of zinc)
Iron	15 milligrams
Magnesium	250–500 milligrams
Vitamin A	25,000 international units
Vitamin C	1,000 milligrams
Vitamin E	400 international units
Zinc	15–30 milligrams

derson, Ph.D., lead scientist in the nutrient requirements and functions laboratory at the U.S. Department of Agriculture Beltsville Human Nutrition Research Center in Maryland and a leading chromium researcher. And although chromium will benefit only those who are deficient, Dr. Anderson reports that most people in Westernized countries receive only 25 percent of the Daily Value of 120 micrograms. So a lot of people are deficient.

Chromium also improves the effectiveness of insulin, the hormone that allows cells to pick up glucose (a simple sugar that your body uses for fuel) from the bloodstream. For this reason, chromium may also be helpful in preventing dia-

Medical Alert

Although vitamins are generally safe, keep these considerations in mind.

- People with diabetes who take chromium should be under medical supervision since their insulin dosage may need to be reduced as their blood sugar levels drop.
- If you have heart or kidney problems, you should talk to your doctor before taking magnesium supplements.
- Vitamin A in the amount recommended here should be taken only under medical supervision, especially if you are a woman of childbearing age. Women who are pregnant should not use this therapy.
- If you are taking anticoagulants, you should not take vitamin E supplements.
- Doses of zinc in excess of 15 milligrams daily should be taken only under medical supervision.

betes, which is common in people who are overweight. People with diabetes who take chromium should be under medical supervision since their insulin dosage may need to be reduced as their blood sugar levels drop.

Doctors who recommend chromium picolinate supplements suggest daily doses ranging from 50 to 200 micrograms. If you'd like to increase chromium through your diet, try whole grain cereals, black pepper, cheeses, and brewer's yeast.

Think Zinc

It's well-documented that zinc—a mineral found in wheat germ, seafood, and whole grains—frequently gets left by the wayside when calorie intake dips below 1,200.

Most experts do not recommend such low calorie regimens. If you're among those who keep a too tight daily calorie tally anyway, you should know that zinc deficiency not only depresses the immune system but also can be a barber's nightmare, causing brittle, dry hair and hair loss.

"When overweight people show any problems with their hair, nails, gums, or skin, I recommend supplementing 20 milligrams of zinc a day," says Dr. Robertson.

Experts usually recommend between 15 and 30 milligrams of zinc daily. Since zinc competes with other metals in the body, however, daily doses of more than the Daily Value of 15 milligrams warrant medical supervision. For the best results, you should take 1 milligram of copper for every 10 milligrams of zinc.

Minerals Make a Difference

Magnesium and iron are the major minerals that doctors find deficient in people who are overweight, particularly in those who are trying to slim down.

Magnesium is essential for every major biological function, including your heartbeat. According to research, even marginal magnesium deficiency is not to be taken lightly, especially when you are dieting and losing weight, as it can lead to potentially fatal heart abnormalities.

"In general, magnesium supplementation helps for a lot of things," says Dr. Steelman. "I use it to treat the muscle cramps that people get when they're trying to lose weight, and it also seems to curb sweet cravings."

Doctors who recommend magnesium supplements call for between 250 and 500 milligrams daily, which is right around the Daily Value of 400 milligrams. (If you have heart or kidney problems, you should check with your doctor before taking magnesium supplements.) Good dietary sources of magnesium include seafood, green vegetables, and low-fat dairy products.

Iron is another frequent victim of low-calorie dieting, says Dr. Steelman. "In fact, it's the most common nutrient deficiency I see, especially in premenopausal women."

The most common complication arising from a lack of iron is iron deficiency anemia, which can cause headaches, shortness of breath, weakness, heart palpitations, and fatigue.

Doctors who recommend supplementing iron suggest 15 milligrams a day, particularly for adults who are following a low-calorie diet to lose weight. To pump some iron into your diet, try steamed clams, Cream of Wheat cereal, tofu, and soybeans.

Calcium is another mineral that's often in short supply in those who are trying to shed extra pounds. Experts suggest making sure that you're getting the Daily Value of calcium, which is 1,000 milligrams; women who are past menopause should aim for 1,500 milligrams daily.

Natural Fat Burner #7: Your Emotions

Like many women who struggle with their weight, Wendy Jarvis traces overeating to an emotional link. In Wendy's case, she says she found herself home alone with "the crazies."

"My husband was at work; my four children were at school," says Wendy, 52, of Devore, California. "Suddenly, I would start feeling insecure and out of control. Then my eating would get out of control, too."

Hershey bars. Milky Ways. Whatever she'd bought for the kids' lunch boxes or for her husband. "It was always chocolate," she says. "Not cake or pies or anything else. I would eat in the kitchen, the living room, the bedroom— all over the house. The more I tried to stop, the more I would eat. That's why I call it the crazies."

Ellie Klenske overate in response to worries about the family business. "There are times in any business when the cash flow is tight," she says. "But when things got stressful, I found myself staring into the refrigerator. And eating."

Frozen vanilla yogurt with nuts, potato chips, or cookies—"always fat-free, of course, but in such copious quantities that it was a lot of calories," says Ellie, also 52, of Redlands, California. "That's why I call food my drug of choice. It's my companion, but it's not necessarily my friend."

Feeding a Deep-Down Hunger

Food is comfort. These days, the emotional impact of food has also become its prime selling point. "We hear about fun-size candy bars, about how making cookies will 'bake someone happy,' and about how chocolate is love," says Susan Moore, R.D., program manager and senior nutritionist of the obesity-management program at George Washington University in Washington, D.C. Small wonder we consume an average of more than 10 pounds of chocolate a year.

Yet if eating becomes your emotional lifeline—a way that you can soothe, cover up, or numb your feelings— then you may find yourself trapped in a vicious cycle of overeating, guilt feelings, and weight gain.

"Everyone does some emotional eating," says Donna Ciliska, R.N., Ph.D., associate professor of health sciences at McMaster University in Hamilton, Ontario, and author of *Beyond Dieting*. "But when a woman overeats for emotional reasons, it becomes a problem."

Emotional eating contributes to excess weight and to the medical conditions that come with unhealthy amounts of body fat, says Dr. Ciliska. If comfort foods like ice cream, chips, chocolate, and pie take the place of healthy edibles in a woman's diet, she is also missing out on vital nutrients that provide optimal energy, prevent disease, and maintain strong bones, she adds. At the same time, it may also indicate that important inner needs are being ignored.

When is emotional eating a problem? When food becomes a distraction, a substitute for love, or even an "anesthesia." When overeating becomes a way to block out anger or depression or to soothe feelings of stress, loneliness, or boredom. These are all signs that your emotions may be a factor in your eating patterns, says Dianne Lindewall, Ph.D., supervising behavioral psychologist of the obesity-management program at George Washington University.

No Comfort in Carrots

Why is it that when that inner voice growls, "Things aren't right—I've gotta eat something!" we're likely to reach for apple pie but not an apple, for carrot cake but not a carrot, for a chocolate milkshake but not a glass of milk?

The answer is simple: Fat- and sugar-laden treats taste good and feel good in our mouths, providing instant pleasure that elevates a bad mood—if only for a few fleeting moments, notes Dr. Lindewall. "On that level," she says, "it's hard for a carrot to compete with a bowl of ice cream."

But our choices of comfort foods are also windows on the past. "One thing we always ask women is, 'What was eating like in your house when you were growing up?'" says nutritionist Barbara Dickinson, R.D., director of nutrition in the Weight Management Center at the Center for Health Promotion and coleader of the Women and Food support group, both at Loma Linda University in California.

"We tend to go for the same kinds of foods and to eat them in the same way—we may overeat because in our families feeling extra-full meant satisfaction," Dickinson says.

Foods like ice cream, cake, and candy are rich in carbohydrates, which may also elevate levels of a feel-good brain chemical called serotonin, temporarily boosting a woman's sense of well-being, says Dr. Lindewall.

This carbohydrate connection may be especially strong for a woman during the second half of her menstrual cycle, after ovulation. At that time progesterone levels rise, causing a drop in blood sugar and increased food cravings, according to Elizabeth Lee Vliet, M.D., founder and medical director of HER Place: Health Enhancement and Renewal for Women in Tucson and Dallas/Fort Worth and author of *Screaming to Be Heard: Hormonal Connections Women Suspect . . . And Doctors Ignore*.

Breaking the Trance: Your Mood–Food Journal

Resisting the siren call of Sara Lee and all the rest requires self-exploration—not sheer willpower.

"The best solution is to cope with the situation that's driving you to eat," says Dr. Lindewall. "And the first step in coping is becoming aware of what's bothering you. Yet instead of putting energy into dealing with the emotional issues, we often avoid them to the point that women tell me they find themselves staring into the refrigerator as if in a trance. They don't know how they got there."

To break the trance, you need to take steps to meet your emotional needs directly, instead of through food. Jot your thoughts in a pocket-size notebook, in your day planner, or on a 3- by 5-inch card. Whatever system you use, the format should be as convenient as possible. That way, you can easily turn to your mood–food journal as soon as you find yourself on the threshold of an emotional eating episode, says Dr. Lindewall.

Use your journal when you feel driven to eat: when you have that sudden, inexplicable urge for a doughnut after a rough morning meeting with the boss, for instance, or when you find yourself reaching into that box of cookies during the lonely hours after dinner. On a blank page or card, answer these questions.

- Am I physically hungry?
- What do I want to eat?
- What am I eating, and how much?
- What am I feeling?
- What am I saying to myself?
- Who is with me?
- What's been going on in the past hours or the past day?

Stress Busters

Skimping on meals raises your risk for a stress-induced feeding frenzy.

"If you aren't eating as much as your body requires, several pressures kick in. Food smells more enticing. It tastes better. Just looking at it makes you want to eat," says Richard Straub, Ph.D., professor of psychology and chairperson of the behavioral sciences department at the University of Michigan in Dearborn. "You can resist these pressures under normal circumstances, but when you throw stress into the mix, you can lose all restraint." In our society, women are even more vulnerable to stress-prone eating than men because women diet more, he says.

How can you stress-proof your eating habits? First, don't diet, says Dr. Straub. Then follow these stress-busting strategies for high-anxiety days.

Schedule stress-reducing breaks. Especially on pressure-filled days, clear room in your schedule for a walk or a talk with a friend, Dr. Straub suggests. "Exercise is especially effective. But talking with someone is also a helpful way to blow off steam."

Try a morning meal. Stress levels rise when your body's low on fuel, says Susan Moore, R.D., program manager and senior nutritionist of the obesity-management program at George Washington University in Washington,

Even if you don't stop eating at first, simply developing the ability to pause before you eat and to identify your true needs—emotional or physical hunger—is a victory, Dr. Ciliska says. "Once you identify the emotions, the long-term goal is finding new ways to cope." Coping could mean anything from trying a new eating plan to learning to ask your spouse for emotional support.

D.C. Some women need more than a bagel and juice for breakfast—a little protein and fat, like a dab of peanut butter, gives you staying power.

Add a snack. Small pick-me-ups at midmorning and midafternoon can keep at bay the low energy that leads to anxiety and stress, says nutritionist Barbara Dickinson, R.D., director of nutrition in the Weight Management Center at the Center for Health Promotion and coleader of the Women and Food support group, both at Loma Linda University in California.

Drink lots of water. Fit in eight 8-ounce glasses of water a day—and drink before you get thirsty, Dickinson suggests. Dehydration can cause headaches and fatigue, so you think you need a snack when all you really need is water.

Go easy on sugar. After eating sugary foods, some women experience reactive hypoglycemia—blood sugar levels rise, then fall dramatically, causing weakness and fatigue, notes Paul J. Rosch, M.D., clinical professor of medicine and psychiatry at New York Medical College and president of the American Institute of Stress, both in New York City.

Think twice about that cocktail. Drinking alcohol is a dangerous substitute for dealing with stressful situations, notes Dickinson. Further, the more you drink, the more excess calories you consume, in the form of alcohol.

Dig for Clues

After keeping a mood–food journal for a week or more, review your notes and search for your emotional eating triggers.

Perhaps you're bored at night and eat for excitement. Maybe you eat after angry arguments with your spouse instead of saying what you feel. Maybe you find yourself in the bathroom, gobbling Twinkies, when your oh-so-critical mother comes to visit. Perhaps you're lonely.

Look for patterns. Your trigger may be a particular feeling or a certain time of day or a high-risk situation, suggests Dr. Lindewall.

Defusing Your Trigger Times

Once you've uncovered your unique triggers, you can take steps to defuse inappropriate eating episodes and meet your emotional needs directly, Dr. Ciliska says. Customize your approach by choosing from among coping strategies that focus on your personal emotional eating issues.

Soothe yourself. As soon as you notice agitated, upset feelings, quickly comfort yourself with a brief, relaxing time-out, suggests Dr. Lindewall. Try a short walk or 5 minutes of deep-breathing exercises, she says.

Think it through. Ask yourself, "What do I need right now?" Try writing your feelings down or calling a friend and talking about what's happening, suggests Dr. Ciliska. Even talking into a tape recorder can help. This step is vital. When you take a moment to sort out what you really need, you reinforce your self-worth and, at the same time, prepare for effective problem solving.

Take action. If you can resolve the issue immediately, do so. You may have to cancel one of two conflicting appointments or make plans to get takeout for dinner on a busy night or clear the air with your spouse, kids, boss, or a coworker, Dr. Lindewall says.

If the issue cannot be resolved immediately, write the solution down and get on with your day. Writing helps clear your head. On the other hand, if you just think about the solution, chances are you'll have trouble getting it out of your mind, she says.

Satisfying Your Emotional Needs— Without Food

As you gain insight into emotional issues that trigger overeating, use the following satisfying strategies to help you nurture yourself and find support. To customize these strategies to your particular needs, experiment to find what works best for you.

Talk about it. Gain new support and learn new coping techniques by sharing your experience with others, suggests Dr. Ciliska. Check with local hospitals or churches to find out about support groups in your area. "In a group, we really find out that we're not alone. It helps with problem solving and getting in touch with emotions," she says. "Behavior change is easier, too."

Self-nurture. Take care of yourself, suggests Dr. Ciliska. You may need more rest, more creative and intellectual stimulation, or the opportunity to express your feelings and have them heard.

You may need new sources of comfort, nurture, and love—like setting aside time for a relaxing bath or listening to your favorite music, or developing new friendships or asking old friends for hugs and attention.

Encourage yourself. Listen to how your self-talk is going throughout the day, Dickinson suggests. Is your inner voice critical or self-defeating or full of commands?

Counter negative messages with truthful, positive responses. For example, turn a comment like "I can't talk to my new coworkers; they won't like me" into "I'd like to get to know them better; I'll begin with some questions about our office during coffee break."

Speak your mind. If you tend to stuff down anger, then learning to ask assertively for what you need can help, Dr. Ciliska says. This may require taking an assertiveness training class, she says.

"I don't know any women, myself included, who haven't benefited from some assertiveness training," notes Dr. Lindewall. "Many times, changing a situation involves dealing effectively with other people. Learning to speak up for yourself without being timid or intimidating is a very important skill."

Make time for simply doing nothing. Stressed? Are mealtimes and snack times the only times you allow yourself to relax? If so, you may be eating just to get a breather from a nonstop routine, notes Sue Irish, a psychotherapist and coleader of the Women and Food support group, sponsored by the Weight Management Center at Loma Linda University.

"A lot of women feel tremendous guilt if they stop working for even a minute," she says. "You work hard all day, eat lunch at your desk, and then spend the evening doing laundry, taking care of the kids, and cleaning the house. You might have a snack or spend a long time over dinner because for most of us it's the only time we give ourselves permission to stop working. Next time, try simply sitting and doing nothing." That could mean listening to music, reading, watching a movie, or simply not doing anything at all, she says.

Put some excitement into your life. Bored? Instead of perking up a dull day with chocolate-covered cherries,

Make Peace with Emotional Eating

Dealing with emotional eating requires solutions tailor-made to your situation. That's what experts like Susan Moore, R.D., program manager and senior nutritionist of the obesity-management program at George Washington University in Washington, D.C., suggest. "Trust yourself to find the best solutions," she says. "And realize that over time you may need new solutions. Constantly adapting is the secret to the mystery of coping with emotional eating."

Exercise is an excellent way to relieve anxiety and boost self-esteem. "It also buys you some time before you eat, time for thinking about what the real issue is and how you can solve it," says Diane Lindewall, Ph.D., supervising behavioral psychologist of the obesity-management program at George Washington University.

Finding special nonfood rewards, like getting a pedicure or buying a new blouse, gives you a well-deserved celebration—without landing you right back in the eat–guilt–eat cycle, says Donna Ciliska, R.N., Ph.D., associate professor of health sciences at McMaster University in Hamilton, Ontario, and author of *Beyond Dieting*.

Finding time for fun fills our human need for play, which serious, responsibility-burdened adults often forget about, says Sue Irish, a psychotherapist who helps lead the Women and Food support group at the Weight Management Center at Loma Linda University in California.

"So often, eating is the only time we let ourselves relax and have a good time," she says. "We forget we need time for recreation."

seek new job challenges, revive a long-lost hobby, or find a new one, suggests Dr. Ciliska.

"I've known people to ask their supervisors for more diverse job responsibilities," she says. "If you feel bored at home, think about past activities you've enjoyed—like a sport or a handicraft." Or peruse the community calendar of your local newspaper for new activities—from volunteer opportunities to quilting circles, tennis classes to wildflower identification walks.

Coping with Comfort Food

Understanding the hot-button issues that push you beyond the comfort zone can take time, says Dr. Lindewall. While you work out better ways to nourish emotional needs, you can also take steps to make your relationship with your favorite comfort foods healthier—and less likely to pack on added pounds or lead to guilty feelings, she says.

Here are some alternative strategies.

Redesign your food environment. Common sense says don't stock up on the high-fat, high-calorie foods. "If you're upset and the only thing available is air-popped popcorn, then eating a lot of that has far fewer calories than, say, premium ice cream or a bag of cookies," Dr. Lindewall says.

Introduce new "convenience" foods. With high-fat fare out of the way, bring in precut vegetables and fruits, suggests Chris Rosenbloom, R.D., Ph.D., associate professor in the department of nutrition and dietetics at Georgia State University in Atlanta. "If you open the refrigerator and find a bowl of sliced peaches, chances are you'll try them," she says.

Eat every 4 hours. Skimping on breakfast and lunch can leave you hungry, irritable, and vulnerable to emotional eating, says Dickinson. The antidote? Eat the right foods, at the right time.

Most people find that a substantial breakfast totaling about 400 calories is helpful, says Moore.

Include a protein food (such as low-fat or skim milk, yogurt, or cottage cheese), grains (like whole wheat toast, oatmeal, or a high-fiber cereal), and fruits, says Dickinson.

"Plan on eating lunch 4 hours later and dinner 4 hours after that," says Dickinson. "Waiting any longer makes most people really hungry. Include foods from at least three of these foods groups: proteins, grains, fruits, and vegetables. It's also good to have a small amount of a healthy fat from avocado, peanut butter, nuts, canola oil, or olive oil. These fats—composed largely of monounsaturated and polyunsaturated fatty acids—help lower blood cholesterol and help make you feel satisfied."

If your stomach growls at midmorning or midafternoon, honor your hunger with a snack such as fruit, low-fat yogurt, or whole wheat crackers and low-fat cheese, she suggests.

Do something with your hands. For some people, unwinding with food can be easily replaced by gardening, a craft, or even computer games—"anything that involves fine motor movement of fingers and hands," says Irish. Somehow small, repeated movements help us chill out after a long day.

"Visualize a spring getting coiled really tight," says Irish. "Everybody gets their internal spring wound up tight all day. Sometimes we eat at the end of the day just to unwind that spring—and it's really the repetitive motion of eating, not the food, that helps us unwind. I play solitaire on my computer, for example. Other people flip through magazines."

Stop, look, and listen. Take a 5- to 10-minute time-out before that first bite and think about what's going on. "Sometimes you just need a few minutes to pull yourself
(continued on page 226)

Are You at Risk for Emotional Eating?

Do you eat when you're blue, angry, lonely, or stressed? Uncovering the triggers that lead to emotional eating could help decipher your eating patterns and resolve the problem of unwanted pounds.

Find out whether—and how much—your feelings rule your food choices with this quiz, developed by Joni Johnston, Psy.D., a clinical psychologist in Del Mar, California, and author of *Appearance Obsession: Learning to Love the Way You Look.* You'll also find advice on unraveling your emotional connections to food. Read the following statements, then rate your own eating habits by using this scoring system.

1 = Never   4 = Often
2 = Rarely   5 = Always
3 = Sometimes

You can tally your score below.

_____ 1. I eat to control stress.

_____ 2. Eating is one of the big pleasures in my life.

_____ 3. I eat well past the point of physical fullness at least two times a week.

_____ 4. When I'm lonely, food comforts me.

_____ 5. I find myself eating to put off things that I don't really want to do.

_____ 6. When my life seems out of control, I have a hard time controlling what I eat.

_____ 7. Sometimes I eat just for fun.

_____ 8. Eating, or trying not to eat, is on my mind a lot.

_____ 9. I eat a lot more when I'm alone than when I'm with others.

_____ 10. Eating soothes me when I feel blue or anxious.

_____ 11. When I was a child, food was a "home remedy" in our house, a source of comfort and love.

_____ 12. Food helps me numb painful feelings and makes me feel better.

_____ 13. When I'm angry, I find myself stuffing the anger down with food.

_____ 14. Sometimes I just can't stop eating.

_____ 15. In a difficult situation, I might retreat and turn to food rather than deal with a problem directly.

_____ Total Score

Scoring: Add up your points for all answers to determine your total score, then read on for the results.

If you scored 15 to 35 points, you have a peaceful relationship with food and are unlikely to routinely respond to difficult emotional situations by eating. Reinforce your healthy attitude by giving yourself weekly self-nurturing treats like a candlelit bubble bath or a massage and by building a strong support system with friends and family. Use relaxation and physical activity to help handle stress. Learning positive coping techniques when life is good keeps the munchies away when times are tough.

If you scored 36 to 59 points, you eat for emotional reasons some of the time. Your eating is sending the message that certain feelings and events in your life need attention. Learn to identify these triggers by keeping a journal of your eating and your feelings. Then develop new ways to relieve stress, fight boredom, or get comfort.

If you scored 60 to 75 points, food has become a major coping strategy—one you probably find less than effective. You have taken the first step toward change by taking this quiz. Now develop a support network or friends and family you can trust to guide and support you in dealing with feelings and food more effectively.

together," says Moore. "You might get a cup of coffee or call a friend. You may be able to identify what's bothering you and decide to put it on the back burner till tomorrow, when you have the time or energy to deal with it directly."

Figure out what you want. If you've paused and still want to nosh, think of ways to minimize the binge. Before you reach for three candy bars or a big slice of cake, be clear about the food experience you're seeking, suggests Moore. "Find out what you really want," she says. "Will a cup of coffee do? Or do you really need a candy bar? Are you looking for a specific taste, or do you want to fill yourself up? If it's a special taste, then maybe a small candy bar is all you need. If it's volume you're after, maybe fruit or popcorn is a smart choice."

Bargain down the size. Once you've decided what you want, ask yourself how much you really need, says Moore. Will one candy bar do, instead of two or three? Will half a piece of cake satisfy you? "By keeping the size down—maybe to just a taste—you control overeating," she says.

Interrupt before the next bite. If you find yourself on automatic pilot, mindlessly reaching into the cookie bag, stop for a moment. "Ask yourself if this is really what you want to be doing and if there is anything else that you'd rather be doing instead," suggests Dickinson. "Often, emotional eating is done quickly. You don't even realize what's going on until the food is all gone. This gives you a chance to pause and be aware."

Balance the calories. Think about how much your indulgence will cost in terms of calories, then plan accordingly. You can compensate for the extra calories that come with an episode of emotional eating by eating less at another meal or two or by getting more physical activity, says Moore.

For example, compensating for a 250-calorie chocolate bar would mean skipping bread and butter at dinner and walking an extra mile.

"If you think about balancing the calories ahead of time, you might decide that the candy bar just isn't worth it," explains Moore. "That's when fruits, and vegetables like baby carrots, start looking really good."

Or you might decide that the candy bar is worth it. "And that's okay," Moore says. "The point is, you're not a bad person for eating this way. You simply have to adjust to avoid gaining weight."

Defuse high-risk times. Your mother's coming for a visit? Almost time for the annual family holiday gathering—and all the tense moments that come with it? "If you can predict high-risk situations and get ready for them, you can balance out the added calories in some way," Dr. Lindewall says. "You can always eat a little less before and afterward."

Challenge all-or-nothing thinking. If you do find yourself crunching instead of coping, don't despair. "That

Lose by Giving

A good way to get inspiration for exercise is to sign up for one of those charity walkathons, run-a-thons, or bike-a-thons. Friends and colleagues agree to donate a certain amount of money depending on how much distance you cover in a given sport. These events benefit a wide range of charities and provide a great source of inspiration for staying in shape, says Ann Marie Miller, exercise physiologist and fitness-training manager at New York Sports Clubs in New York City.

Miller has discovered that helping out a favorite charity and getting exercise are not the only benefits to be gained from participating in one of these events. "It also makes you grateful that you have a healthy body that can exercise," she says.

doesn't make you a bad person or mean that you've ruined everything," says Dickinson. "Even if you still experience some overeating, remember that you're making a change. It takes time. Don't lose sight of that."

When Overeating Gets Totally Out of Control

"The binge eaters who come to us for treatment are often women over 35 who seek solace by eating large quantities of food and who feel out of control during a binge," says Marlene Schwartz, Ph.D., codirector of the Center for Eating and Weight Disorders at Yale University.

During a binge, a woman often chooses foods that she regards as forbidden or dangerous or fattening—chips, or slice after slice of toast slathered with peanut butter. She may feel as if she's in a trance.

Unlike women with bulimia, another behavioral problem, binge eaters do not purge afterward, Dr. Schwartz says. And unlike women who overeat once in a while, binge eaters are caught in a cycle that repeats itself several times a week.

"This isn't the same as eating too much at Thanksgiving dinner," Dr. Schwartz says. "Women with this condition have usually binged at least twice a week for at least 6 months. Food has become a way to cope, but then it ends up making them feel worse about themselves."

Bingeing or Simply Overeating?

Researchers are still debating the best ways to tell whether a woman has binge-eating disorder. But, they say, you may have binge-eating disorder, and not a simple overeating problem, if you frequently eat abnormally large amounts of food, if you feel unable to control what or how much you eat, and if you also have at least two of these experiences or feelings during a binge:

- Eat more rapidly than usual
- Eat until uncomfortably full
- Eat alone or in secret
- Feel depressed, guilty, or ashamed afterward

Another way to check is by asking yourself these four questions. If you answer yes to two or more, you may have binge-eating disorder, says Denise Wilfley, Ph.D., director of the Center for Weight Control and Eating Disorders at San Diego State University and the University of California, San Diego.

1. Are there times during the day when you could not have stopped eating even if you wanted to?
2. Do you ever find yourself eating unusually large amounts of food in a short period of time?
3. Do you ever feel extremely guilty or depressed afterward?
4. Do you ever feel even more determined to diet or to eat healthier after the overeating episode?

Biggest, Baddest Bingeing Triggers

What prompts a binge? Loneliness, anger, sadness, frustration, and stress are often the triggers, Dr. Schwartz notes. Dieting, or severely restricting certain foods, can also lead to a binge episode.

"A woman who takes care of everything else in her life—her children, her spouse, her job, and her home—may not take the time to take care of herself. She may not feel entitled to put her own needs on the front burner," Dr. Schwartz says.

A woman may feel uncomfortable about conflict and find it easier to sweep her feelings under the rug, rather than share them with the people she's close to, Dr. Schwartz says. Or she may simply be so busy that she has no time to sit down and sort out uncomfortable emotions.

And so she eats. She may hide the evidence or even stay home from social engagements, work, or school in order to eat.

"Bingeing soothes bad feelings temporarily by numbing you out," says Dr. Wilfley. "But afterward a binge eater feels worse and tries to punish herself. She may resolve not to eat at all the next day or to severely restrict certain foods."

But inevitably she does eat again—either for emotional reasons or hunger or in response to the lure of forbidden food. "It's a natural reaction to eat when hungry," Dr. Wilfley says. "But just by eating, a woman who binge-eats may feel that she has blown her diet. She feels bad. So she eats more. And so the cycle of bingeing begins again. In this way, dieting and restricting foods can actually lead to more binge eating."

Breaking Free

If you have, or suspect you have, binge-eating disorder, Dr. Wilfley says that you can overcome it by discovering and meeting your own emotional needs and by developing the habit of eating regular meals and snacks.

"A woman can try self-help techniques," Dr. Schwartz says. "Then, if she finds that she's not able to make changes on her own, finding a therapist or a support group is an excellent idea."

Here are ways to begin helping yourself overcome this disorder.

Write it all down. Keep a mood–food journal, as you would for simple emotional overeating. Use it to monitor all the foods you eat. Note when and how much you eat and how you were feeling at the time, suggests Dr. Wilfley. You may find that you skip meals, then binge out of hunger, or that certain situations trigger emotions that lead to bingeing.

Stick with regular meals and snacks. That means eating breakfast, lunch, and dinner as well as snacks in between to ward off hunger, Dr. Wilfley says. Follow this schedule even if it means having a meal soon after a binge, she says.

"After a binge, work even harder to get back into a regular schedule, rather than deprive yourself," she says. "You might have a small dinner if you binged beforehand, but the idea is to slowly become accustomed to regular eating and get out of the cycle of getting most of your calories from binges and little energy or nutrition from regular meals."

Worried about weight gain? In reality, your weight will probably stay the same or even drop as normal eating patterns replace high-calorie binges.

Put your needs first. The same steps toward self-esteem that help women overcome emotional eating are vitally important for women with binge-eating disorder, says Dr. Wilfley. So remember to take time to nurture yourself, challenge critical self-talk, and ask for what you need from others in an assertive way.

Problem-solve. Once you've identified your personal trigger emotions and situations for binge eating, try to spot them before a binge begins. Then consider and evaluate solutions other than food. You may feel lonely, for example, and could call a friend, watch TV, or go for a walk. After considering some alternatives, act on your best solution.

Reach out. Many women find that a therapist or a support group is invaluable in making the journey beyond binge eating, Dr. Wilfley says. "Just remember that this condition is just gaining recognition. Be sure to ask any therapist or group leader you're considering about their experience in treating binge-eating disorder."

To find a support group for eating disorders, contact your local hospital. The staff may also be able to refer you to qualified therapists. For a list of university-based eating disorder treatment centers, contact the Weight-Control Information Network, run by the National Institutes of Health, at 1 WIN Way, Bethesda, MD 20892-3665.

Natural Fat Burner #8: Prayer

When she was 35, Carre Anderson of Westerville, Ohio, was trying a new diet nearly every week. Most of them tried to change what she ate. Yet none forced her to confront her growing love affair with food. "I was constantly organizing, planning, and scheming to make sure that I got enough to eat," says the stay-at-home mother of three.

Years of this behavior left Anderson frustrated and extremely overweight. Although she's only 5 feet 5 inches tall, Anderson tipped the scales at 217 pounds.

Finally, her failure to handle her eating drove her to her knees to pray for help. Soon after, the wife of the pastor of her church invited her to preview a videotape for a faith-based weight-loss study program that the church was considering.

While watching the video, Anderson was transfixed. "The Bible verses convinced me that I was dealing with more than just an issue of controlling the food."

Anderson joined the church study group and adopted its principles. The result? In one year, she lost 100 pounds.

And not only has she kept the weight off for a year, but she now leads the church weight-loss group as well.

Eating for the Wrong Reasons

Can praying and reading Scripture really help someone lose weight? Gwen Shamblin, R.D., author of *The Weigh Down Diet* and founder of the Weigh Down Workshops, one of the most popular faith-based weight-loss programs, says yes, because it sets the right priorities.

"Diets make the food 'behave.' But it's not the food's fault," says Shamblin. Instead, she believes that overeating is caused by a deep-seated spiritual emptiness. "We have two empty needing-to-be-fed holes in our bodies," Shamblin says. "One is the stomach, and the other is the heart."

And when we don't get the love, acceptance, and approval that we need to fill our hearts, some of us try to fill it up with food. "The term that I use for this is emotional eating," says C. Dwight Bain, a Christian counselor and regional communications director in Orlando for New Life Clinics, the largest provider of Christian-based counseling in the United States. "Say something happens at work that makes me mad. If I think that there's nothing I can do about it, I'll go home and eat and eat and eat. I'm not eating out of hunger or any physical desire. I'm eating because I'm upset."

In fact, "a high percentage of eating disorders like anorexia, bulimia, and overeating have a direct correlation to biochemical depression," says Jacqueline Abbott, Dr.P.H., codirector of the Kartini Clinic for Disordered Eating in Portland, Oregon. Biomechanical depression occurs when we have a deficiency in the naturally occurring chemicals in the brain.

One of the most common symptoms of depression is unhealthy eating habits, says Dr. Abbott. "It could be not wanting to eat or, more likely, eating all the time in an attempt to help soothe or calm yourself," she says.

Some of us get so fanatical about our love of food, it borders on worship. "We dress for it, putting on stretch clothes to make sure that there is nothing coming between us and that binge," says Shamblin. "We plan a secret rendezvous with food all day long. Thinking about it, anticipating it, buying it, cooking it, smelling it—all our senses are alive for it."

We soon discover, though, that overeating doesn't satisfy our emotional hunger and leaves us worse off than when we started. "It robs us," says Shamblin. "It robs us financially. It robs us of our clothing. It robs us of our self-esteem. It robs us of relationships. It robs us of our freedom. And so we wake up and realize that our health is bad—mental health and spiritual health. Our souls are empty. We're longing. We're hurting."

Getting It Right

Instead of turning food into a god, Shamblin says that we need to worship the true God. "We need to quit making rituals of this stuff. Take the time and energy and love for food or anything else that is a strong hold and give it back to God," she recommends.

"We are talking about healthy eating and regular exercise, as opposed to compulsive overeating," says Bain. "We are talking about freedom from food."

Here are some suggestions on how to put food in its rightful place in our lives.

Study someone thin. One quick way to get insight into how obsessed we are with food is to observe the role that it plays for someone who is lean and healthy and has been for most of her life. Shamblin says that she did this when she had a weight problem, and she was shocked. In the time that it took her to gobble a full fat-laden meal at a fast-food restaurant, her thin friend had barely eaten half of a hamburger. And then her friend had the nerve to start wrapping up the rest to take home! "This was a real eye-opener," she says.

Respond to the signals. Forget diet shakes, fat-loss pills, and fat-free products. Shamblin says that the best way to lose weight is by responding to your body's true signals of hunger and fullness. True hunger, she says, "is a rumbling, a growl, that's felt at the top of the stomach under the sternum." And true fullness is "a polite feeling—we're simply no longer hungry."

When our bodies signal that we're truly hungry, we should eat, and we should stop when it says that we're full, suggests Shamblin. This may mean that we eat one large meal a day or small meals five or six times a day, depending on what's right for our bodies.

Often, people eating this way discover that their volume is reduced to about one-half to one-third of what they used to eat. "That automatically decreases fat intake by about 50 to 75 percent," says Shamblin.

Slow down. Eating more slowly allows the food time to hit the bloodstream, which in turn allows blood sugar levels to rise, triggering the brain's appetite center and producing a feeling of fullness so that we don't overeat, says Elizabeth Lee Vliet, M.D., founder and medical director of HER Place: Health Enhancement and Renewal for Women in Tucson and Dallas/Fort Worth and author of *Screaming to Be Heard: Hormonal Connections Women Suspect . . . And Doctors Ignore.*

Breaking food into smaller pieces, taking smaller bites, getting involved in conversation while we eat, and stopping for a minute or two during our meals all can help, Shamblin says.

Enjoy it. We should give thanks for each and every bite. And savor them, allowing them to melt in our mouths.

Take emotional pain to God. If we're having problems at work or in our relationships or if we're feeling emotional or spiritually barren, we shouldn't turn to snacks. We should turn to a higher power.

Beat back binges with prayer. And when a binge really hits? "We should cry out to God and say, 'God, what I'd really like to do is finish off all the cheese dip and chips and the rest of the gallon of rocky road ice cream. Don't let me. Make me feel better than a binge,'" says Shamblin.

Join a group. Whether it's the Weigh Down Workshop or one like it, getting involved in a weight-loss group can help improve your chances of success during those first, crucial months, says Bain. "A lot of people who have struggled for years with weight problems wonder, Can I do this? That's where resources and people in a weight-loss group can step into the gap early on and help out."

Natural Fat Burner #9: Visualization

If you can think it, you can do it. Sound too simplistic? It's not.

When you visualize an action, you engage 80 percent of the neural pathways that are used in actually performing the action, says Howard J. Rankin, Ph.D., psychological advisor to the TOPS (Take Off Pounds Sensibly) Club and author of *Seven Steps to Wellness*. Just by picturing yourself thinner or envisioning yourself exercising and eating better, you are already 80 percent on your way there.

Take this classic visualization example: Imagine sucking on a lemon. Before you know it, your salivary glands kick in, as if an actual lemon were in your mouth. Your mind persuades your body that you taste a lemon, and it acts accordingly, says Emmett Miller, M.D., medical director of the Cancer Support and Education Center in Menlo Park, California, creator of the *Imagine Yourself Slim* relaxation/visualization audiotape, and author of *Deep Healing*.

Use this phenomenon to your advantage. Through visualization, your mind can convince your body that you are thinner, stronger, faster, and younger so that you act in a way that leads to being thinner, stronger, faster, and younger.

"When an image is created in a deep state of relaxation, it serves as a strong autosuggestion," Dr. Miller says. "There is a real tendency of the mind and the nervous system to do all those things that would bring about that image."

The Art of Weight-Loss Visualization

With visualization, you picture as reality the positive result—what you want to achieve. It provides a clear, defined goal and the path to get there. So if you're not yet seeing the results you want in the mirror, take another look—this time with your imagination.

"People tend to focus on what they don't like and what they fail to do, instead of getting a clear picture of what they want," Dr. Miller says.

There are three styles of visualization to help you with your weight-loss goals: visualization as motivation, visualization as a coping technique, and visualization as a stress reliever. No matter which style you use, keep in mind the three basic tenets of successful weight-loss visualization.

Wade into the deep end. To truly visualize for weight loss, it helps to be in a relaxed, calm, and thought-free state, especially at first. "Deep relaxation eliminates distracting thoughts. If not in a relaxed state, people have a tendency to think negative thoughts. But being relaxed allows the message to affect you more powerfully," Dr. Miller says.

Before doing a visualization exercise, try the following relaxation response. Find a comfortable, quiet place to sit. Close your eyes as you relax all your muscles, beginning with your feet and moving up toward your face, says Dr. Miller. Breathe in through your nose. Say the word *one*, or any word that relaxes you, with each exhale.

Think details, details, details. Don't just visualize yourself as slim. Picture the definition and the shape of your finely tuned muscles. Imagine the colors, textures, and patterns of a favorite outfit that you want to wear. The more realistic your vision, the more real it will be, Dr. Miller says.

Experience your vision, right down to your senses. This is not a game where you pretend to be someone else. When you visualize, you should be able to *feel* what it is like to be a thinner, younger you. Smell, hear, touch, and taste your vision. "The more senses that you can bring into it, the better," Dr. Miller says.

Picture This: A Thinner, Motivated You

An Olympic skier closes her eyes and sees herself maneuver and master the course. She pictures each turn, each hill, each bump in the mountain. By the time she actually skis, she has completed her run a thousand times in her mind. Then the fun part: She visualizes herself up on that podium, accepting a gold medal and hearing the national anthem play as she enjoys the spoils of her success.

You, too, can use visualization just as elite athletes do. By seeing yourself as thinner, you ingrain in your mind the idea of what you want—and the actions that you have to take to get there. "By picturing yourself with a slim body, you'll find that your appetite will decrease, your desire to exercise will increase. You'll start doing the things that will bring about your image," Dr. Miller says.

Also, your image serves as motivation. You will see and feel what it's like to be a thinner, younger you. Tasting that success—even if it is through a mental image—en-

The Power of Affirmations

Affirmations are positive statements that help change negative, unhappy emotional and mental states, says Susan Lark, M.D., a physician in Los Altos, California. Here are some of her recommended affirmations. To do the affirmations, sit in a comfortable position and repeat each statement three times, slowly and clearly.

- My mood is calm and relaxed.
- I handle stress easily and effortlessly.
- I feel wonderful.
- I am enjoying my life more and more.
- My life brings me pleasure.

courages you to keep at it, even during the tough times. "The brain likes when you show it a goal," he adds.

For support and motivation, you should visualize once or twice a day, Dr. Miller says. It takes 10 to 15 minutes each time for beginners. As you progress, you'll be able to use these visualization techniques in 5 minutes whenever you need to.

Before you begin, find a picture—perhaps an old photo of yourself or one from a magazine—that represents what you want to look like. Pick a realistic one. "It's good to have a picture of the body you want," he says.

To start, go into a state of deep relaxation, then use the following as a visualization guide. If you have trouble employing the technique during a state of deep relaxation, make an audiotape to guide you through, or buy a guided-imagery tape, Dr. Miller suggests.

Your body. Picture how you want your body to look. Notice the definition of your muscles. Also focus on particular body parts—your thinner waist, your toned chin, your shapelier and firmer legs.

Your clothes. Visualize yourself in a specific outfit, one that you have always wanted to wear. See yourself in this outfit in your thinner, lighter, but also stronger body. Feel the fabric against your skin and feel how the clothes hug your body. Imagine every detail: the color, style, cut, and pattern.

Your look. What does the new you look like? Picture your new haircut, new makeup, new accessories. See yourself shopping for new clothes, picking out styles that you might not have worn before.

Your actions. What do you want to do with this new body? See yourself walking farther and faster or taking up new activities, like jogging, biking, or waterskiing.

Your reactions. Hear the compliments people will shower on you: "You look fabulous!" "You've lost weight!" "How did you do it?" See their faces as they admire your new look. See your face as you beam with delight.

See Past the Roadblocks

Just as elite athletes visualize their paths to success and envision their victories, they also picture the obstacles that pop up. They think about what may block their way, and then they visualize how they will overcome it.

You can use visualization in the same way for weight loss. Picture something that would normally lead you astray, then see yourself rise above that problem.

Basically, visualization acts as a fire drill, Dr. Miller says. "Now everybody knows the exits. You are much more ready to handle it when it happens to you. The correct response has been programmed in beforehand."

To use visualization as a coping or problem-solving technique, go into deep relaxation. Then think about the situation step-by-step, visualizing the minutest details. Make it as real as possible, which will increase the chance that when faced with the predicament, you'll react just as you had imagined, Dr. Miller says.

You may have your own personal circumstances that you want to visualize, but there are some that almost all people trying to lose weight want to overcome. Here are Dr. Miller's suggestions to steer your way clear from temptation.

The buffet. Picture yourself walking up to the buffet table. Imagine what you take: a skinless piece of chicken breast; a side of broccoli; a whole wheat roll; a salad of lettuce, tomatoes, onions, and peppers covered in a light vinaigrette; and perhaps some strawberries for dessert. Watch yourself put the spoon down as you take small, reasonable portions. Pass over the candied yams, the cream sauce, the desserts. Walk away from the buffet as soon as you have what you want. Imagine how satisfied and happy you are with your food choices and how good it feels to push your plate away. Savor feeling full but not stuffed.

The saboteur. A friend offers you chocolate chip cookies. You say, "No, thank you." But she persists and tests your will by saying, "This one time won't hurt you" or "Oh, come on, don't ruin the fun." Look her straight in the eye and say, "I am in the process of choosing my food carefully, and I would appreciate your support on this by not offering, suggesting, or giving me food." Smile because you know that you successfully defeated a temptation. And imagine how good you feel physically, because you didn't eat the cookies, and emotionally, because you didn't give in to someone else's demands.

The fast eater. Imagine sitting down at the table. Take a good, long look at your plate. Savor the colors: the golden yellow of the corn, the deep green of the asparagus, the bright red of the tomato. Study each grain of rice, noticing the shape and texture. Smell the aroma, taking a minute to enjoy each food's distinct bouquet.

Finally, take your fork and pick up a small amount of food. As you bring it closer to your face, smell the food again. Put it in your mouth, but don't chew. Let the food sit on your tongue for a moment. Then begin to chew, and roll the food around your mouth and tongue, touching all the different tastebuds. Chew the food at least 25 times, enjoying every second of flavor. After you swallow, take another moment to enjoy what you just ate. Take a sip of water. Begin the process again.

The exercise skipper. See yourself putting on your sneakers, anticipating your daily walk as a time of relaxation and fun. Picture your surroundings as you walk and imagine how the brisk air feels on your face. You grow stronger and leaner with each step. Visualize your lungs taking in the air and breathing it out without effort. Imagine how far you can walk and how good you feel afterward.

Take a Mental Vacation

Study after study has shown that stress is the number-one reason people fail to keep off weight. When you're faced with stress, your body often wants to reject all that is good for weight loss, so you wind up making bad food choices and skipping exercise.

But with visualization, you can short-circuit that response without endangering your progress. "When you use imagery, you develop a sense of mastery and control over your own circumstances," says Stephan Bodian, former editor of *Yoga Journal* and author of *Meditation for Dummies*. Stress-release visualization triggers your body to respond as if it were on vacation—tension slips away, breathing becomes slow and relaxed, and your mind lets go of all distractions.

Try one or all of the following visualization techniques to ease tension and reduce stress.

- Imagine taking a warm shower, Bodian says. As the water falls around you, feel it wash away all your worries, problems, and concerns.
- Imagine warm honey melting from the top of your head, Bodian says. It slowly covers your body, flowing down until it completely envelops you. Allow the warm, thick liquid to absorb all your tension and stress.
- Picture yourself at your favorite getaway: a beach, the woods, the mountains. Imagine every aspect of the experience, says Kolleen Biel, program manager at the New Albany Health and Wellness Center in New Albany, Ohio. For example, if your dream spot is the beach, imagine seagulls flying overhead, smell the salt in the air, hear the gentle crashing of the waves, feel your toes sink into the cool sand beneath your feet.
- Think of something that you love to do: gardening, doing needlepoint, reading a book, watching your favorite TV show, sitting in a beloved overstuffed chair, Biel says.
- While under stress, take a second and say, "My mind is clear and relaxed. My muscles are loose and relaxed." Just the power of suggestion relieves stress and tension, Biel says.

Fat Finder's Guide

This handy guide will help you start identifying how many grams of fat are in the foods you eat. If you don't see specific foods you eat on this list, check the labels or pick up one of the many handy paperback books listing fat-gram counts.

Food	Portion	Fat (g)
Breads and Bread Products		
Breads		
Italian	1 slice	0
Pita	1	0.6
Cracked wheat	1 slice	0.9
Mixed grain	1 slice	0.9
Rye	1 slice	0.9
White	1 slice	1.0
Pumpernickel	1 slice	1.1
Whole wheat	1 slice	1.1
Oat bran	1 slice	1.2
French	1 slice	1.4

Food	Portion	Fat (g)
Crackers		
Rye wafer	1	0
Whole wheat, low sodium	1	0
Rye snack	1	0.4
Wheat snack	1	0.4
Graham	1	1.3
French toast		
Frozen	1 slice	5.0
Homemade	1 slice	6.7
Muffins		
English	1	1.1
Oat bran, with raisins	1 small	3.0
Blueberry	1 small	4.0
Corn	1 small	4.0
Bran	1 small	5.1
Pancakes and waffles		
Waffles, frozen	2 (2.5 oz each)	7.0
Plain pancakes	4 (4")	7.6
Buckwheat pancakes	4 small	8.0
Rolls and biscuits		
Brown-and-serve roll	1	2.0
Hard roll	1	2.0
Hamburger/hot dog bun	1	2.1
Biscuit	1 small	5.1
Others		
Melba toast	1 piece	0
Matzo	1 piece	0.3
Rice cake	1	0.3
Corn tortilla	1	1.1
Bagel	1	1.4
Taco shell	1	2.2

Food	Portion	Fat (g)
Cereals		
Wheat flakes	1 cup	0
Corn squares	1 cup	0.1
Puffed rice	1 cup	0.1
Puffed wheat	1 cup	0.1
Farina	1 cup	0.2
Shredded wheat	1 biscuit	0.3
Bran flakes	1 cup	0.7
Cornflakes	1 cup	0.7
Wheat germ, toasted	1 Tbsp	0.8
Raisin bran	1 cup	1.0
Bran squares	1 cup	1.4
Oat rings	1 cup	1.5
Oatmeal, instant	1 pkg	1.7
Oatmeal, cooked	1 cup	2.4
Wheat germ, toasted	½ cup	6.1
Granola	1 cup	33.1
Condiments		
Horseradish	1 Tbsp	0
Soy sauce, low sodium	1 Tbsp	0
Teriyaki sauce	1 Tbsp	0
Worcestershire sauce	1 Tbsp	0
Cranberry sauce	¼ cup	0.1
Dill pickle	1 med.	0.1
Ketchup	1 Tbsp	0.1
Sweet pickle	1 small	0.1
Sweet relish	1 Tbsp	0.1
Tamari	1 Tbsp	0.1
Yellow mustard	1 Tbsp	0.6
Brown mustard	1 Tbsp	1.0
Green olives	5	2.9
Tartar sauce	1 Tbsp	8.0

Food	Portion	Fat (g)
Dairy Products and Eggs		
Cheeses		
Yogurt cheese	1 oz	0.6
Cottage cheese, 1% fat	½ cup	1.2
Parmesan, grated	1 Tbsp	1.5
American, singles	1 oz	2.0
Swiss, diet	1 oz	2.0
Mozzarella, skim-milk	1 oz	4.5
Cottage cheese, 4% fat	½ cup	4.7
Blue cheese	1 oz	4.9
Ricotta, part-skim	¼ cup	4.9
Feta	1 oz	6.0
Monterey Jack, light	1 oz	6.0
Mozzarella, whole milk	1 oz	6.1
Swiss	1 oz	7.8
Brie	1 oz	7.9
Ricotta, whole milk	¼ cup	8.0
Monterey Jack	1 oz	8.6
American, processed	1 oz	8.8
Colby	1 oz	9.1
Cheddar	1 oz	9.4
Cream cheese, regular	1 oz	9.9
Eggs		
White only, raw, large	1	0
Whole, raw, large	1	5.0
Milk and cream		
Evaporated skim	½ cup	0.3
Skim	1 cup	0.4
Nondairy whipped topping, frozen	1 Tbsp	0.9
Nondairy creamer	1 Tbsp	1.0
Half-and-half	1 Tbsp	1.7

Food	Portion	Fat (g)
Buttermilk	1 cup	2.2
Low-fat, 1%	1 cup	2.6
Sour cream, imitation	1 Tbsp	2.6
Cream, light	1 Tbsp	2.9
Sour cream, cultured	1 Tbsp	3.0
Low-fat, 2%	1 cup	4.7
Cream, heavy, whipping	1 Tbsp	5.5
Whole, 3.3%	1 cup	8.2
Evaporated whole	½ cup	9.6

Yogurt

Plain, fat-free	1 cup	0.4
Plain, low-fat	1 cup	3.5
Plain, whole	1 cup	7.4

Desserts and Snacks

Cakes

Angel food	1 slice	0.1
	(2 oz)	
Sponge	1 slice	3.1
Strawberry shortcake	1 slice	8.9
Pound	1 slice	9.0
	(1 oz)	
White, with chocolate icing	1 slice	11.0

Candies

Chocolate fudge, plain	1 oz	2.9
Milk chocolate, with almonds	1 oz	10.1
Milk chocolate, with peanuts	1 oz	10.8

Cookies and brownies

Gingersnap	1	0.6
Vanilla wafer	1	0.9

Food	Portion	Fat (g)
Desserts and Snacks (cont.)		

Cookies and brownies (cont.)

Food	Portion	Fat (g)
Fig bar	1	1.0
Chocolate chip	1	2.2
Chocolate/vanilla sandwich	1	2.3
Brownie, with chocolate icing	1	5.0

Cupcakes

Food	Portion	Fat (g)
No icing	1	3.0
Devil's food, with icing	1	4.0
Chocolate, with icing	1	5.0

Doughnuts

Food	Portion	Fat (g)
Plain	1 (2 oz)	10.8

Frozen desserts

Food	Portion	Fat (g)
Fruit-flavored frozen yogurt	½ cup	1.0
Orange sherbet	½ cup	1.9
Vanilla ice milk	½ cup	2.8
Vanilla ice cream	½ cup	7.2
Vanilla ice cream, premium	½ cup	11.9

Pastries

Food	Portion	Fat (g)
Apple turnover	1 oz	4.7
Eclair, with custard and icing	1	13.6
Cheesecake	1 slice	16.3

Pies

Food	Portion	Fat (g)
Apple	1 slice	13.1
Custard	1 slice	14.0
Blueberry	1 slice	15.0
Chocolate cream	1 slice	15.1
Pecan	1 slice	27.0

Food	Portion	Fat (g)
Pudding and gelatin		
Gelatin	½ cup	0
Vanilla pudding, sugar-free, 2% milk	½ cup	1.2
Chocolate pudding, sugar-free, 2% milk	½ cup	1.9
Chocolate pudding	½ cup	4.0
Tapioca pudding	½ cup	4.0
Rice pudding, with raisins	½ cup	4.1
Vanilla pudding	½ cup	5.0
Custard, baked	½ cup	7.5

Dips and Dressings

Food	Portion	Fat (g)
Dips		
Clam, garlic or French onion	1 Tbsp	2.0
Guacamole	1 Tbsp	2.0
Jalapeño or green onion	1 Tbsp	2.0
Bacon and horseradish	1 Tbsp	2.5
Dressings		
Italian, no oil	1 Tbsp	0
Sweet and sour	1 Tbsp	0.3
Blue cheese, low-fat	1 Tbsp	0.9
French, low-calorie	1 Tbsp	0.9
Italian, low-calorie	1 Tbsp	1.5
Mayonnaise-style	1 Tbsp	5.2
French	1 Tbsp	6.0
Ranch-style	1 Tbsp	6.0
Italian, regular	1 Tbsp	7.1
Blue cheese	1 Tbsp	7.6
Russian	1 Tbsp	7.6
Vinegar and oil	1 Tbsp	8.0
Thousand Island	1 Tbsp	8.1

Food	Portion	Fat (g)
Fats and Oils		
Butter		
Whipped	1 tsp	2.4
Regular	1 tsp	3.8
Margarine		
Corn oil, diet	1 tsp	1.9
Whipped	1 tsp	2.7
Corn oil, stick	1 tsp	3.8
Corn or safflower oil, soft	1 tsp	3.8
Mayonnaise		
Low-calorie	1 tsp	1.3
Regular	1 tsp	3.7
Oils		
Olive	1 tsp	4.5
Vegetable	1 tsp	4.5
Fruits and Juices		
Dried fruits		
Dates	½ cup	0.4
Prunes	½ cup	0.4
Raisins	½ cup	0.4
Figs	½ cup	1.2
Fresh fruits		
Grapefruit	½ med.	0.1
Grapes	10	0.1
Peach	1 med.	0.1
Casaba melon, cubed	1 cup	0.2
Figs	2 small	0.2
Honeydew melon, cubed	1 cup	0.2
Orange, all varieties	1 med.	0.2

Food	Portion	Fat (g)
Papaya, cubed	1 cup	0.2
Kiwifruit	1 med.	0.3
Apricots	3 med.	0.4
Cantaloupe, cubed	1 cup	0.4
Apple, with peel	1 med.	0.5
Banana	1 med.	0.6
Blueberries	1 cup	0.6
Mango	1 med.	0.6
Nectarine	1 med.	0.6
Strawberries	1 cup	0.6
Bartlett pear	1 med.	0.7
Pineapple, cubed	1 cup	0.7
Raspberries	1 cup	0.7
Sweet cherries	10	0.7
Watermelon, cubed	1 cup	0.7
Plums	2 med.	0.8
Florida avocado	1 med.	15.4
California avocado	1 med.	30.0

Juices

Cranberry	1 cup	0.1
Prune	1 cup	0.1
Grape	1 cup	0.2
Apple	1 cup	0.3
Orange	1 cup	0.5

Gravies and Sauces

Gravies

Beef, canned	¼ cup	1.2
Turkey, canned	¼ cup	1.2
Mushroom	¼ cup	1.6
Chicken, canned	¼ cup	3.6

Food	Portion	Fat (g)
Gravies and Sauces (cont.)		
Sauces		
Chili	¼ cup	0
Tomato, canned	¼ cup	0.1
Barbecue	¼ cup	1.2
Taco, canned	¼ cup	1.4
Marinara, canned	¼ cup	2.1
Spaghetti, canned	¼ cup	3.0
White, thin	¼ cup	4.9
White, medium	¼ cup	7.8
White, thick	¼ cup	10.6
White, very thick	¼ cup	13.5
Legumes		
Beans		
Mung, sprouted	1 cup	0.2
Lima, boiled	1 cup	0.5
Navy, cooked	1 cup	1.0
Red kidney, canned	1 cup	1.0
White, small, boiled	1 cup	1.2
Refried	1 cup	2.7
Chickpeas, canned	1 cup	4.6
Others		
Lentils, boiled	1 cup	0.7
Peas, split, dried, cooked	1 cup	1.0
Meats		
Beef		
Bottom roast, lean	3.5 oz	9.6
Arm pot roast	3.5 oz	9.9

Food	Portion	Fat (g)
Rib roast, lean	3.5 oz	13.7
Blade pot roast	3.5 oz	15.2
Hamburger, extra lean	3.5 oz	16.0
Hamburger, lean	3.5 oz	18.4
Salami	3.5 oz	19.9
Lamb		
Rib chop, lean, broiled	1	7.4
Leg, lean, roasted	3.5 oz	7.7
Shoulder, lean, roasted	3.5 oz	10.7
Pork		
Canadian bacon	1 slice	2.0
Tenderloin roast, lean	3.5 oz	4.8
Ham, extra lean	3.5 oz	5.5
Ham roast	3.5 oz	8.9
Loin roast, lean	3.5 oz	13.5
Shoulder roast	3.5 oz	14.9
Chop, lean, broiled	3.5 oz	15.2
Italian sausage links	1½ (3.5 oz)	17.2
Bologna	4 slices (3.5 oz)	19.7
Loin roast, lean and fat	3.5 oz	21.5
Chop, lean and fat, broiled	3.5 oz	27.0
Sausage patties	4 (3.5 oz)	30.9
Sausage links	8 (3.5 oz)	32.4
Veal		
Shoulder and arm roast, lean	3.5 oz	5.8
Rib, lean, braised	3.5 oz	7.8

Pastas and Grains

Food	Portion	Fat (g)
Pastas		
Whole wheat macaroni, cooked	1 cup	0.8
Spaghetti, cooked	1 cup	1.0

Food	Portion	Fat (g)

Pastas and Grains (cont.)

Pastas (cont.)

Spinach pasta, cooked	1 cup	1.3
Egg noodles, cooked	1 cup	2.0
Chow mein noodles	1 cup	11.0

Grains

White rice, cooked	1 cup	0
Bulgur, cooked	1 cup	0.4
Brown rice, cooked	1 cup	1.8
Spanish rice, cooked	1 cup	4.2

Poultry

Chicken

Breast, no skin, roasted	3.5 oz	3.5
Thigh, no skin, roasted	1 small	5.7
Chicken roll, light meat	3.5 oz	7.3
Breast, with skin, roasted	3.5 oz	7.8
Leg, no skin, roasted	3.5 oz	8.0
Leg, no skin, stewed	3.5 oz	8.1
Breast, floured, fried	3.5 oz	8.8
Thigh, floured, fried	1 small	9.2
Breast, batter-fried	3.5 oz	13.1
Leg, roasted	1 small	15.4
Dark meat, with skin, roasted	3.5 oz	15.8
Salad	3.5 oz	17.5

Duck

No skin, roasted	3.5 oz	11.1
With skin, roasted	3.5 oz	28.2

Food	Portion	Fat (g)
Goose		
No skin, roasted	3.5 oz	12.6
With skin, roasted	3.5 oz	21.7
Turkey		
Breast, no skin, roasted	3.5 oz	0.7
Turkey loaf, from breast	3.5 oz	1.6
Smoked	3.5 oz	3.9
Turkey ham, from thigh	3.5 oz	5.0
Dark meat, no skin	3 oz	7.2
Turkey pastrami	3.5 oz	7.2
Turkey roll, light meat	3.5 oz	7.2

Nuts and Seeds

Food	Portion	Fat (g)
Chestnuts, roasted	½ cup	0.9
Sesame seeds, roasted	1 Tbsp	4.3
Pumpkin/squash seeds, roasted	½ cup	6.0
Cashews, oil-roasted	½ cup	31.4
Cashews, dry-roasted	½ cup	31.8
Pistachios, dry-roasted	½ cup	33.8
Almonds, dry-roasted, whole	½ cup	35.6
Peanuts, oil-roasted	½ cup	35.7
Sunflower seeds, dried	½ cup	35.7
Spanish peanuts, dried	½ cup	35.9
Filberts (hazelnuts)	½ cup	36.0
Pecans	½ cup	36.6
Persian/English walnuts	½ cup	37.1
Brazil nuts	½ cup	46.4
Macadamia nuts	½ cup	49.4

Food	Portion	Fat (g)
Seafood		
Finfish		
Anchovy, fillet, canned	1	0.4
Tuna, light meat, canned in water	3.5 oz	0.5
Cod, cooked	3.5 oz	0.9
Haddock, cooked	3.5 oz	0.9
Flounder, broiled	3.5 oz	1.5
Sole, broiled	3.5 oz	1.5
Red snapper, cooked	3.5 oz	1.7
Halibut, broiled	3.5 oz	2.9
Rainbow trout, cooked	3.5 oz	4.3
Swordfish, cooked	3.5 oz	5.1
Pink salmon, canned	3.5 oz	6.0
Bluefin tuna, cooked, dry heat	3.5 oz	6.2
Salmon, cooked	3.5 oz	7.5
Tuna, canned in oil, drained	3.5 oz	8.1
Sardines, canned in tomato sauce	3.5 oz	11.9
Mackerel, cooked	3.5 oz	17.6
Shellfish		
Shrimp, cooked	3.5 oz	1.1
Scallops, steamed	3.5 oz	1.4
Clams, cooked	3.5 oz	5.8
Scallops, breaded, fried	3.5 oz	11.4
Shrimp, breaded, fried	3.5 oz	12.1
Vegetables		
Carrot, raw	1 med.	0.1
Celery	1 stalk	0.1
Romaine lettuce	1 cup	0.1
Sweet potato, baked	1 med.	0.1
Zucchini, boiled	1 cup	0.1
Butternut squash, baked	1 cup	0.2

Food	Portion	Fat (g)
Cauliflower, raw	1 cup	0.2
Potato, baked, no peel	1 med.	0.2
Spinach	1 cup	0.2
Acorn squash, baked	1 cup	0.3
Mushrooms	1 cup	0.3
Sweet pepper	1 small	0.3
Tomato	1 med.	0.3
Broccoli, boiled	1 cup	0.4
Cabbage, boiled	1 cup	0.4
Green beans, boiled	1 cup	0.4
Asparagus, boiled	1 cup	0.6
Summer squash, boiled	1 cup	0.6
Brussels sprouts, boiled	1 cup	0.8
Corn ear, fresh, boiled	1 small	1.0
Onion ring, fried	1	3.0
French fries, frozen	10 pieces	4.4
Hash-brown potatoes, frozen	½ cup	9.0
Potato salad, homemade (eggs and mayonnaise)	½ cup	10.3

Index

Underscored page references indicate boxed text.